WHAT IS THE SAFEST, MOST SATISFYING WAY FOR YOU TO HAVE YOUR BABY?

The Birth Primer is the only book that explains to parents all the birth options available to them. It describes all the current childbirth methods now being used, including the nonmedicated or "natural" approaches of Lamaze, Bing, Dick-Read, Leboyer, and others. It summarizes the many procedures used in medicated births, including spinal, caudal, epidural, Caesarian, forceps, fetal monitoring, and labor inducement. It also discusses father assistance, birth attendance by labor coaches, and the role of midwives—as well as examining the respective advantages of having your baby at the hospital, home, maternity center, or clinic. It documents the experiences of other parents, and the opinions of experts and institutions from all areas of the obstetric community. There's also a full reference list of childbirth education associations, preparation manuals, and books on childbirth.

But, most important, *The Birth Primer* will give you the feelings as well as the facts connected with giving birth—to assure that this special moment in your life be as beautiful and rewarding as possible.

THE BIRTH PRIMER

SIGNET Titles of Special Interest to Parents

THE BIRTH PRIMER

A Source Book
of Traditional and Alternative Methods
in Labor and Delivery

Rebecca Rowe Parfitt

Foreword
by
John B. Franklin, M.D.

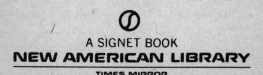

A SIGNET BOOK
NEW AMERICAN LIBRARY
TIMES MIRROR

The ideas, procedures and suggestions contained in this book are not intended as a substitute for consulting your physician. All matters regarding your health require medical supervision.

The publisher wishes to thank the following for permission to reproduce photographs or extracts:

Figures 1–7 (pp. 12–15): Reproduced with permission from the *Birth Atlas,* published and copyrighted by Maternity Center Association, N.Y., N.Y.
Photos p. 16, p. 170 (by Paco North), & p. 185 (by Ed Lettau): Reproduced with permission, courtesy of Maternity Center Association, N.Y., N.Y.

(The following page constitutes an extension of this copyright page.)

Published by arrangement with Running Press.

 SIGNET TRADEMARK REG. U.S. PAT. OFF. AND FOREIGN COUNTRIES
REGISTERED TRADEMARK—MARCA REGISTRADA
HECHO EN CHICAGO, U.S.A.

SIGNET, SIGNET CLASSICS, MENTOR,
PLUME and MERIDIAN BOOKS
are published by The New American Library, Inc.,
1633 Broadway, New York, New York 10019.

First Signet Printing, February, 1980

1 2 3 4 5 6 7 8 9

PRINTED IN THE UNITED STATES OF AMERICA

Premise

One day in the winter of 1976, Chuck Deal, printer, friend, and the father of a newborn, came into our publishing offices to discuss a printing problem. In the course of some social chatter, he mentioned the frustration which he had gone through in trying to find an appropriate book that would explain all the possible birth procedures that he and his wife, Jayne, could choose from. Chuck had searched the shelves of two public libraries and every bookstore in his community, but could find no single volume that explained all the options available to them. He and Jayne finally went through the process of reading a handful of childbirth books and ultimately decided upon a father-assisted delivery. Chuck suggested that someone ought to publish one resourceful volume that would present the full range of alternatives and enable prospective parents to make initial decisions and then guide them to the best books, organizations, and appropriate segments of the medical community. The author spent a year gathering material and writing the book that Chuck Deal was looking for, but could not find. . . . We call it *The Birth Primer*.

RUNNING PRESS

Contents

Foreword

There is a new appreciation of birth that is well worth telling. After a century of deliveries based on fears for the mother and her baby and avoidance of pain at almost any cost, we are beginning to see births focused on the great value of the mother's and father's love. With all its senses the newborn baby responds to loving attention. A little understanding is required, but all of us can attune our senses to those of the baby. The quiet revolution in the delivery room has been to recognize that after securing a live birth, those who would help the parents must aid and encourage those vital emotional transactions which flow back and forth between the parents and the newborn. This emotional flow finds ready expression in breast feeding. It is the physical representation of the emotional. By complex sucking the baby transmits its thought and feeling; by cuddling and nourishing, the mother transmits her complete response to her baby.

The identification of these bonds of love coincides with a growth of medical attention in the problems of the past. This attention was based on the realities of miscarriage, stillbirth, prematurity, and congenital malformations. While miscarriage and malformations may be destined from the earliest divisions of the fertilized egg, stillbirth and prematurity are now regarded as potentially preventable by medical intervention. Even with congenital malformations parents can be offered early termination of a pregnancy which they may regard as unsupportable. The medical intervention consists of asking the baby: "Are you all right?" and "Will you be all right for the time remaining?" Some real success has been in the prevention of infant death during labor, but the greatest success has occurred in preventing the death of very premature infants. The success of neonatologists working in intensive care nurseries has been such that reorganization of obstetric care is taking place. Babies carrying special risks are now delivered at hospitals with such nurseries.

The new efforts in medicine to prevent needless infant

death are costly. In addition to high financial costs, in some instances these efforts appear to prevent the attachment of parents to their babies. New mothers are easily discouraged. Pediatricians have learned that mothers of premature babies, when separated from them, act as if the baby were dead even when the baby is surviving perfectly. Premature babies have experienced a higher degree of child abuse. Consequently the intensive care nurseries work from birth to involve the parents. Some neonatologists feel that breast milk is mandatory for premature babies and encourage mothers to touch and feed their tiny infants. In obstetrics the barriers are less obvious, and obstetric interference with mother-child attachment is just beginning to be examined. It is clear, however, that high costs, the failure to share planning with patients, and arbitrary hospital regulations have fostered a growing mistrust of obstetricians and hospital-based delivery.

This mistrust has accompanied a rejection of a materialistic technology which has failed to prevent wars and eliminate poverty, and which stifles human feelings. Faith in man has been replaced by a faith in nature. If only we do not interfere with what nature has intended for us, we can enjoy the unlimited goodness of life. What is overlooked is the essential randomness of biologic events. People's bodies and their babies come in different shapes and sizes. Incredibly small shifts in development may produce a beautiful baby with a hopeless circulation.

Because medicine often ignores feeling, alternatives have appeared. If one feels impassioned by natural beauty and makes love in such a setting, why not deliver there? More appropriate, perhaps, one may want a warm, dark place, soft and secure, in which to have a baby. A small but significant number of people—parents, midwives, doctors—are contributing to these childbirth alternatives. Some are trying to document their safety; others talk about the wonderful shared experience.

Finally, we have come to recognize that childbirth is not something that can be repeated many times. Too many pressures exist to curb family size. At the same time our individualism has led us to want the most out of each life experience. The potential for personal growth in pregnancy, delivery, and child nurture is unparalleled.

This mix of personal biologic and medical goals produces a tension that can be reduced by a clear stating of the facts.

Rebecca Parfitt has presented both the facts and the feelings of childbirth without overstating either. She captures vividly some of the anger people have felt toward medical intervention, and she presents fairly the problems that can justify it. She directs the reader to the many sources of help. No longer does one rely on a single person or a single book. For the pregnant woman and the expecting couple, *The Birth Primer* describes the many aids in childbirth: reading, classes, films, groups, hospitals, and birth alternatives.

As a physician I believe that I am in partnership with the parents for a common goal. This book does much toward the understanding of that goal.

HBFranklin MD
Philadelphia

JOHN B. FRANKLIN, M.D.

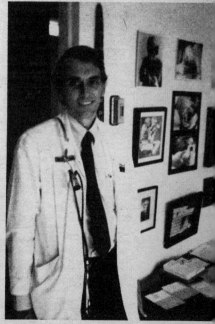

John B. Franklin, M.D., is Medical Director at Booth Maternity Center in Philadelphia, Pennsylvania. He is also Assistant Professor of Gynecology and Obstetrics at Thomas Jefferson University, Philadelphia. Dr. Franklin received his medical degree from Vanderbilt University Medical School in 1958.

1

Labor

The way we give birth to our young is that the muscular organ in which the offspring has been nurtured for nine months begins to contract. The contractions work to open the neck of the uterus and then expel the baby and the nourishing organ down the birth canal and out through the vaginal opening. This process, which pushes the baby out of its warm, wet, nearly dark, and rhythmically rocking home is as complicated a physical drama as humans are likely to be able to witness. At the same time, it is a simple miracle. We call it labor.

The term labor should be understood to *include* delivery; the actual birth of the baby is followed shortly after by the expulsion of the placenta, the third and final stage of the process. Labor is work, and it is hard work. Labor is an end to pregnancy and a beginning for a new human life in a newly-shaped family.

This chapter describes the course of a "typical" labor. Although no two experiences of labor are ever quite the same, a familiarity with the basic process, its vocabulary, and the sensations and emotions which others have felt can serve as a source of confidence and relaxation for an expectant mother (and her partner) in the managing of her own (or their own) labor. Following this account is a description of variations and complications we sometimes encounter in the birth-giving process. The chapter also includes a brief account of several facets of the postpartum period.

BEGINNING OF LABOR

Labor begins approximately 266 days after conception, or 280 days after the first day of the mother's last menstruation. This 280-day term is often viewed as ten lunar (28-day) months, a period which fits neatly with the lunar character of the menstrual cycle. Obstetricians and midwives most often chart the progress of the pregnancy in weeks, 40 in all. The fetus is halfway to maturity at 20 weeks. Another popular way to divide the nine months is into thirds, three trimesters of about 13 weeks each.

1

It is wise to compute your due date. This will help you keep track of the developments in your pregnancy. Also, should there be a need for medical procedures during your labor, the medical team assisting you might need to know how mature your unborn baby is. (Quick calculation of the due date can be made using Ely's Table, found in the Appendix of this book.)

Though it may occasionally seem endless to you, these 280 days are a short time for all the growth that has taken place. We all originate from two cells—sperm and ovum—joined. The fertilized egg duplicates itself, dividing into two cells; these follow suit, and so on, until a pin-point-size mass attaches itself to the lining of the uterus about one week after fertilization. About 39 weeks later, a human being is born.

At term, a baby is usually 19 or 20 inches long, curled up to about 14 inches, and weighs on the average 7 to 7½ pounds. She swallows the water (amniotic fluid) surrounding her, urinates, hiccups, twitches, kicks, sucks a thumb from time to time, may scratch herself with fingernails, hears, and has open eyes which can see in a pale glow during late pregnancy when the tissues between her and the source of light are sufficiently thinned out for stretching. She alternates periods of waking and sleeping, holds on the cord, and waits.

Figure 1 shows the fetus at term, at completion of pregnancy, ready for labor. The uterus sits low in the pelvic basin, very much stretched out. In non-pregnant times this muscle is about the size of a small grapefruit; now it measures about 10 inches by 14 inches. Within the uterus is the semitransparent membrane sac of amniotic fluid. Salty and almost clear, this fluid is our first environment. (Salt water is deeply familiar to us; earliest life arose from the primeval oceans, after all, and every cell inside the body actually floats in salt water containing both dissolved nourishment and cellular waste—an environment not unlike that which the fetus floats in.) Amniotic fluid, like other aspects of the intra-uterine life, is a marvel of accommodation and adaptation. It serves the growing fetus in a number of ways: the fetus drinks it, urinates into it, and practices moving around in it. It is a valuable cushion, serving as a shock absorber when contractions begin to push the fetus against the not-quite-opened cervix. During labor the fluid distributes the pressure equally within the uterus.

Attached to the uterine wall, on the left in Figure 1, is a spongy mass which is also connected to the fetus, via the umbilical cord. This is the placenta, a remarkable liverlike organ which has served as the nourishment center for the growing fetus. Food and oxygen, the substances necessary for life, come via the mother's blood, into the placenta, through the vein in the cord, and into the fetus. Then blood containing carbon dioxide and other waste flows from the fetus through the arteries in the cord, to the placenta where it transfers the wastes to the mother's circulation. Then the fetal blood is resupplied with oxygen and nutrients. The placenta is the key coordinator of all metabolic exchanges between mother and fetus.

The cord is about 20 inches long, an inch-and-a-half thick (there is quite a bit of variation), pale blue, and covered with a tough membrane; it contains the one vein and the two arteries.

The placenta and cord are the fetus' life line, the soil, roots, and stem of the human plant in *utero*.

Figures 1 through 7 are plates from a large spiral-bound book called the *Birth Atlas*, an internationally appreciated childbirth education aid. The *Birth Atlas* photos are of a sculpture series presented by the Maternity Center Association at the World's Fair in 1939-1940 in New York. Life-size plaster sculptures form this series, showing the growth of the fetus during gestation (pregnancy) and the stages of labor.

By looking at these and at drawings you can get a feel for the nature of the vaginal route to extra-uterine life: short, but tricky, with several bony obstacles and a descending, then ascending, pattern. It is none too roomy either; the fetus is compressed, must twist and turn.

There sits the baby, ready to make the journey. It is a trip usually requiring many hours. In pre-surgical times a difficult labor could last days. The shortest labor I ever heard of was one and one-half *minutes*. An "average" labor for a woman having her first baby (she is called a *primapara*) is 12 to 14 hours; for a woman giving birth to a second or subsequent child (a *multipara*), it is given as 7. Modern obstetrics tends to apply the ancient rule of thumb that the sun should not set twice on the same labor. Long labors are those reaching 24 to 30 hours, by which time a standard hospital or a maternity center would be seriously considering intervention, as would most birth attendants in a home setting. Recent research has determined that 11 to 15 hours is optimal length—long enough for the stretching out of the tissues that need to stretch and long enough for the fetus not to be traumatized, but also short enough so that maternal fatigue does not start to create stress for the baby.

It is not understood what actually starts labor. Dr. Leboyer points out in *Birth Without Violence* that at the time of Hippocrates in ancient Greece it was believed that the fetus demands to be born. It gets cramped in there and the food is pretty skimpy toward the end, so the child simply propels itself out into the world. Leboyer comments that modern science is coming to support this view. In a way, it is.

In the modern obstetrical view of how labor gets started, there are two main components: the hormonal and the mechanical. One theory (Benson, 1976) states that the mother, the fetus, and the placenta all contribute to the maintenance of pregnancy. When the fetus reaches maturity, certain ''restraints'' are removed, triggering contractions of the uterus. These signals about maturity and restraint are sent among the mother, fetus, and placenta via *hormones*.

Hormones are chemical substances created in ductless organs of the body and released directly into the bloodstream (this is the body's endocrine system). Hormones regulate growth and cell activity all over the body. Progesterone and estrogens are the hormones which affect sexuality and reproduction. Progesterone does seem to have a stabilizing, antiexcitatory function. During pregnancy it inhibits uterine contraction, protecting the fetus from untimely expulsion. At the same time estrogens are increasing the contractility of the uterus. From the seventh month of pregnancy on, research suggests, secretion of estrogen outweighs secretion of progesterone, bringing on more and more emphatic contractions.

Then there is the mechanical aspect. The uterus becomes more excitable and contractile simply from being stretched out, while the fetus is large enough to be exerting downward pressure. The mother is certainly aware of this as she searches for a comfortable sleeping position at the end of pregnancy and finds herself constantly going to the bathroom as the growing baby crowds all the organs in the pelvic region.

Furthermore, the *presenting* part of the fetus—that is, the part most down into the pelvis, the part (usually the head) that will come out first—is putting pressure on the cervix, irritating it and starting to stretch it out. An increase in this stretching of the cervix, combined with an increase in secretion of the hormone oxytocin and an increase in contractility of the uterus, all work together in a positive feedback cycle.

Whatever the physiological chain reaction, the time does arrive when you become aware that you are in labor. Some advance notice may come your way if you experience diarrhea for a few days. When labor is imminent, diarrhea may sometimes serve the body by relieving the pressure for space in the pelvis.

A signal for some women that labor will begin within hours, or at most, a day or two, is the passing out through the vagina of a small amount of mucus, the plug which has helped seal the cervix closed for these months. The mucus is often flecked with blood; hence its name, *bloody show* (or just *show*). Its passing continues for some women throughout first-stage labor.

Sometimes the thin membrane sac bursts, another sign of the onset of labor. This occurs because of the pressure against it, causing the amniotic fluid to come gushing or trickling out, warm and salty. This is called the breaking of the bag of waters, or the rupture of the membranes. The quality of the amniotic fluid is of great interest to doctor and midwife: usually it is clear, but a fetus in distress will sometimes relax the bowels *in utero*, staining the fluid with meconium, which is the technical name for the contents of the fetus' intestinal tract. Meconium gives a greenish or brownish cast to the waters; if your waters are thus colored, you should immediately tell the doctor or midwife about it. Often, however, the membrane, which is like plastic wrap, doesn't break until the baby starts to move down the birth canal.

FIRST STAGE: OPENING UP

Early

Early first-stage labor involves slow, muscular contractions to the point where the neck of the uterus is opened about 4 centimeters wide.

Indeed, contractions are the most reliable sign that labor has begun. A *contraction* is, literally, a drawing or pulling together. When you flex your biceps or make a fist, the fibers of the relevant muscles are pulling together, shortening, squeezing, temporarily clamping down on the blood vessels. When your calf muscle cramps in a charleyhorse you are experiencing a muscle contraction that is involuntary. Such is the uterine kind.

The uterus, after all, is an organ of muscles, three interlaced sets of them. Its muscular structure is explained by Dr. Grantly Dick-Read, author of *Childbirth Without Fear*, in a way that helps to give a picture of what the work of labor entails.

The uterus consists of three separate kinds of muscles. The muscle of the outermost layer runs longitudinally, that is, up and down, and is concentrated mostly in the upper part of the uterus, called the fundus (in any organ the part that is farthest from the opening is called the fundus). The work of this set of muscles is to pull up, shorten and tighten, and push the baby down.

The middle layer is a mass of muscle in which the blood vessels are located; this muscle contracts to squeeze the blood out of the uterine wall, then relaxes and lets the blood vessels fill up again.

The inner layer goes around the uterus in a circular, lateral way, and is found almost exclusively in the lower, cervical end of the

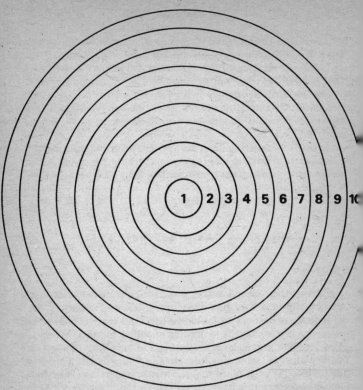

Dilatation Chart, actual size. Sometimes a midwife will hold up such a chart for a laboring woman to give her a sense of how far along she is in the opening up of the cervix. Dilatation is measured in centimeters. Complete dilation is 10 cm.

uterus. These muscles maintain the uterus in its closed up state; when they contract, as in a frightened, tense woman, they are keeping the cervix extra tight. Thus, explains Dr. Dick-Read, the laboring woman's ability to relax will prevent this layer of muscle from tightening up and so reduce the painful conflict with the opening-up action of the outer layer.

Contractions originate from the outer musculature around the top portion of the uterus. The contracting motion moves downward, becoming weaker. The uterus contracts intermittently in a rhythm that soon establishes itself as unique to you. Individual contractions have a characteristic wavelike shape, starting low, building to a peak about halfway through, and then declining. The contractions of the different stages of labor feel different, and have different functions.

The painless contractions during late pregnancy are called Braxton-Hicks contractions (after a 19th-century English gynecologist). These usually intensify as labor approaches; they are, in fact, beginning the work of labor. The cervix is closed tight throughout pregnancy. For the baby to get out, the cervical opening must soften (become "ripe," as they say), and its sides must be taken up. This ripening process is called *effacement*. With a first baby, effacement is usually complete before cervical opening up, or *dilation*, begins. In a multipara, effacement and dilation occur more or less simultaneously. It is this process which constitutes the body's task in first-stage labor: to gradually open up the cervix, making the uterus and the birth canal continuous. From Figures 1, 2, and 3 you can see how this progresses.

In the primapara each part of the labor is longer than in the multipara. First stage in a primapara lasts, on the average, 12 to 14 hours; in a multipara, more like 6 or 7. During this time the cervix stretches from being closed to being dilated 10 centimeters (cm), the largest dimension of the head of most babies. Midwives usually measure dilation in fingers' worth, 2 cm per fingers; so if you are fully dilated you are 5 fingers dilated. Complete cervical dilation is the job of the first stage of labor.

The mother's task in first-stage labor is to facilitate the opening-up process by relaxing and by keeping the oxygen supply adequate. When the body is in a relaxed state, the uterus is aided by not having to compete with other muscles for the mother's blood supply. Doctors and midwives universally report that a woman who is able to relax during first-stage labor shortens that process, to the benefit of both baby and mother. Each contraction compresses the baby's space and temporarily cuts down his/her oxygen supply. Deep, relaxed breathing, staying upright, and moving around moderately help maintain a good oxygen supply for mother and fetus. When you lie flat, the blood return through the vena cava is reduced by the weight of the uterus, reducing the speed at which the blood supply is re-oxygenated.

Active

At about 4 cm of dilation the labor feels as if it is in earnest. Contractions at this point are usually regular, about 5 minutes apart, and last 45 seconds or so. Labor now is referred to as active, and if you are going to a hospital or maternity center, this is when you would probably choose to go. Many women find their faces flushing around this time. The relaxed, deep breathing that keeps early contractions under control usually is not adequate for relieving discomfort after 5 or 6 cm of dilation, and a quicker, panting rhythm takes over (see Chapter 2).

Transition

Most women consider the last 2 or 3 cm of dilation the toughest part of labor. This is the transition period, the final phase of the opening up of the cervix.

The contractions are stronger, longer, and closer together during transition than during any other part of the labor. "Hurricane hour" is a good description I have heard. Contractions build quickly to an aching intensity and hold for 90 seconds or more; barely a minute later another one starts. They seem to come piggyback. Most women find that contractions establish their own rhythm—one gigantic, two minor, one gigantic, for instance.

Other signs that you are in transition include nausea, trembling, and chills. The physical sensations of transition often cause a woman to feel overpowered, engulfed, absorbed in her task, unable to converse, panicky, irritable. It is a time for the support person to be doubly encouraging and understanding; it is no time to be alone. "You know," my neighbor Connie related, "I was eighteen when Krissie was born, and it turned out she was a breech, coming out rear first, and back then, well, we didn't know, we were just kids really, and there I was alone, and there's that fear, you know, the feeling of 'I might die.' And there's that sense, underneath the fear, the sense of being swept up in a force of nature so powerful that your ordinary experience of your self is gone."

Every woman's transition is unique to her. Estelle, in Raven Lang's *Birth Book,* speaks of transition: "Now I started to get a bit worried. I remember that the flowers in my garden began to look a little mean. . . ."

It is genuinely helpful to know that the titanic contractions of transition are a brief phase. The control they require (not to tense up, especially) and the stress they put on the baby, whose whole environment is violently squeezing and tumbling him/her around, could not be borne by anybody for long. It has been estimated that even in a primapara transition lasts only 9 to 12 contractions—one hour perhaps.

If a woman is inclined to be as little medicated as possible, but feels that transition is altogether too much, she might well be able to stay with it if someone with close, loving support were to say, "How about just lasting through another handful of these—the hardest part is short—you can do it!'' or something to that effect. It really does help to remember that these contractions are finite in number, to take each one as it comes.

The pressure put on the mother's lower abdomen by the more and more deeply engaged head begins at the end of transition to give the mother a feeling of needing to push. You can hear a catch in the breath of a woman experiencing this urge; it is very powerful.

But if the woman pushes before the cervix is opened up enough to accommodate the infant's head, she is, in effect, battering the baby's head against the cervix. This is particularly rough on the baby if the fluid cushion is already gone; moreover, the mother is needlessly tiring herself in the bargain. Midwife or doctor can assure the woman—and so can her support person—that she should resist the urge to push until told to do so. This is hard. A similar restraint will be asked one other time during labor, just before the baby's head comes out, to ease the baby out gently. This kind of restraint is exquisitely difficult. Imagine exerting control over a strident call of nature, such as the need to do a bowel movement or the urge to vomit. Imagine that in a barrage of physical sensations you will find the will to breathe with a blowing out and a panting, to *not* push, to *not* give in to the demand from your body.

Once the transition contractions have completed their work by bringing you to 10 cm dilation, the toughest stage of labor is done.

SECOND STAGE: PUSHING THE BABY OUT

Early

At last the cervix is open, gone; the uterus and the birth canal are continuous, and labor is in a new phase, the second stage, where you get to push the baby out. Figure 3 illustrates full dilation, the continuity between uterus and birth canal.

It takes a few contractions in the second stage to get the hang of pushing. Having practiced a comfortable upright or semi-upright position and a useful breathing pattern (see Chapter 2) can help get this expulsion effort underway. Your companions will see the baby's head at the vaginal opening, just a small patch, a dime's worth, they say, at the height of a push, then it recedes. The baby is inching its way down the birth canal, propelled by the combined push of the mother's effort and the contractions of the uterus.

These contractions are very different in character from transition contractions. There is more time between them, and the painful stretching of cervical tissue is over. You work *with* these contractions, relaxing the perineum (stretch of tissue between the vagina and anus), bearing down, pushing the baby down and out. A midwife or support person can help remind you of your task, here and throughout.

This stage is as short as a handful of contractions for a mother who has given birth before. The primaparous mother may be in second-stage labor for 45 minutes to 2 hours. It is exciting and exhausting work. The effort of it is like pushing a grand piano across a large warehouse floor alone. For most mothers this stage is the most rewarding part of labor, a real relief.

The birth

Finally the patch of baby head that shows with the pushing does not recede between pushes, meaning that the baby has overcome the last major obstacle, getting over the pubic bone. The head is *crowning*. The whole perineum will be bulging, accompanied by a burning, tearing sensation. If the midwife or doctor and you have decided to wait and see if an episiotomy (cut to enlarge the opening) is necessary or not, this is the moment of decision. If the perineal tissue is stretching gradually, and is not shiny and thin, which would indicate it could stretch no more, you may be able to forego the little cut. Massage at this time by one of the attendants can help to prevent cutting or tearing. And your control—pushing when told and pausing when your attendant says not to push—is crucial.

The perineum, like a turtleneck sweater, shrinks over the baby's crowning head. The new body is tightly compressed, leading usually with the back of the head, while the chin is down toward the chest. The head emerges, rotating; then the shoulders; then the rest of the baby slips out. There's a sudden and tremendous relief of pressure when the baby comes out. To me it felt like a "popping" sensation. Then the wait and answers to questions: is the baby a girl or a boy? Is the baby all right? The attendant will usually remove the mucus and other obstructing fluid from the nose and mouth of the baby, using a bulb syringe.

Many undrugged babies let out a yell even before they are fully born; the cooler air of the delivery room or wherever you are (perhaps under a sequoia, like one West Coast story I heard) is almost sure to be cooler than the 99 or so degrees Fahrenheit of the uterine environment. This temperature change can shock the newborn's system into beginning its new respiration on the spot.

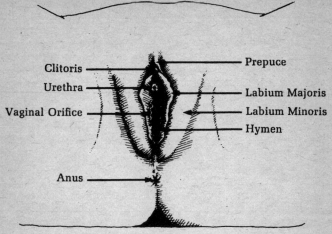

Surface view of the perineum, the stretch of tissue between the vaginal opening and the anus. The perineal area is also called the pelvic floor.

Usually, however, the baby comes out a purplish lump of a person, not breathing (oxygen still comes via the cord), wrinkled, and often still covered with vernix, the waxy substance which has protected the skin of the fetus during these nine underwater months.

The cord

In about 25% of births the umbilical cord is wrapped around the baby's neck at birth: after the head comes out, the cord usually can be slipped around and off. If the cord is too tight, the accoucheur (attendant) will have to clamp and cut it immediately, before allowing the mother to complete delivery. But usually, when the baby comes out, mother and child are still connected umbilically; and the baby's supply of oxygen is still obtained via the blood in the umbilical cord, which after birth is still connected with the placenta. And the placenta, at the end of second-stage labor, is yet attached to the wall of the uterus.

At the time of birth the cord contains as much as 100 cc of blood, or about one-third the total blood supply of the newborn. As Constance Bean points out in *Labor & Delivery,* postponing the clamping and cutting of the cord for a few minutes to allow this blood to drain into

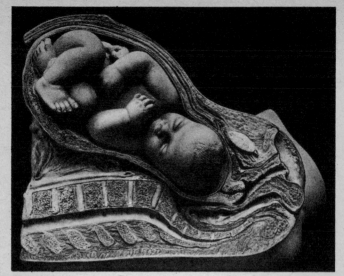

Figure 1 *Before Labor Begins. This baby is well developed and in the most usual position, head down and facing the mother's right side. The cervix is long and thick.*

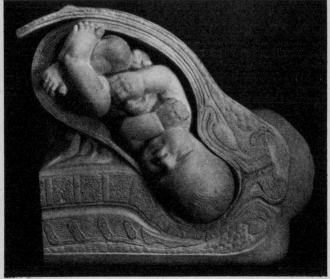

Figure 2 *First Stage Labor. The baby has descended into the pelvic cavity. The cervix is completely effaced and has begun to open up (dilate).*

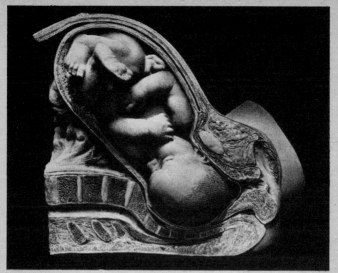

Figure 3 *Full Dilation, Beginning of Second Stage Labor. The baby has turned and is moving down. The membranes, still intact, are bulging in front of the baby's head.*

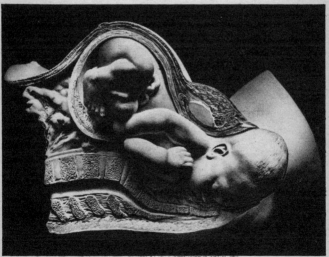

Figure 4 *Crowning of Baby's Head. The membranes have ruptured, the perineum is bulging. The crown of the baby's head can be seen at the vaginal opening. The baby's face is turned completely toward the mother's back.*

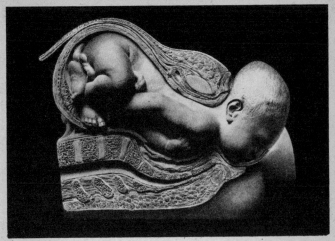

Figure 5 *Near the End of Second Stage. The baby's head emerges; the perineum is shrinking. The baby's head turns upward.*

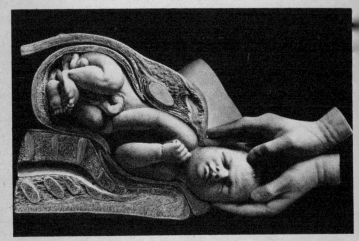

Figure 6 *Birth. The baby's head turns as it is being born, and the shoulders rotate.*

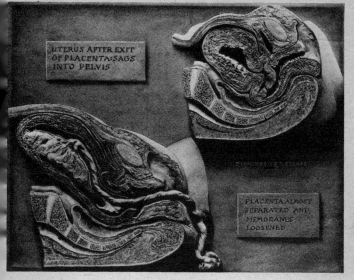

Figure 7 *Third Stage. Placenta, on the left, is separating from the wall of the uterus. After it is expelled, the uterus sags into the pelvis until continuing contractions begin the process of returning it to its pre-pregnant state.*

the baby's system helps prevent anemia in the newborn and helps prevent heavy bleeding in the mother. Dr. Leboyer also advocates postponement of cord clamping or cutting, though his emphasis seems to derive mostly from impassioned respect for the child. He wishes that our obstetrical practices be guided by a heightened sense of concern for the infant; and so he reminds us of the shocking suddenness of the change which the newborn must make in order to fill his new lungs with air for the first time and begin respiration. The more gradual the transition from dependent to independent respiration, suggests the author of *Birth Without Violence*, the more humane and less traumatic will be the experience for the astonished neonate. This placental transfusion (i.e., complete drainage of the cord's arterial blood into the baby) requires perhaps seven minutes at the most.

Further: a leading obstetrical textbook, *Williams Obstetrics, Fifteenth Edition*, reports on research from the early sixties which shows that too-early clamping may be a factor in the development of respiratory distress syndrome in the newborn.

At home births fathers often cut the cord, usually waiting, I would wager, until the cord has ceased to pulse and has turned from purplish to pale.

For Native Americans still maintaining their traditional ways, as for many peoples of the world, cord-cutting is an important ceremonial occasion. There will be a traditional cord-cutting implement of a particular material—an obsidian knife, perhaps, or a seashell—to be wielded by a designated person, at the appropriate moment.

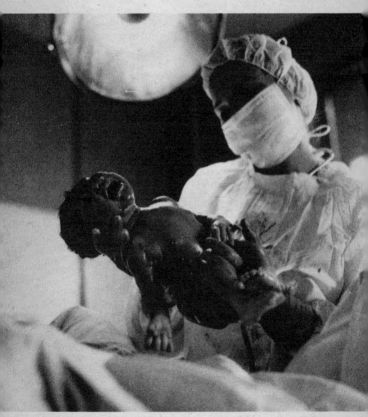

Immediately After Birth. This baby, still connected to the placenta via the cord, is taking a first breath of air. A nurse-midwife is in attendance.

THIRD STAGE: THE AFTERBIRTH

The work of the placenta is done. The uterus continues to contract after the baby is out; these contractions squeeze and shake the placenta loose from its mooring on the endometrium (see Figure 7). Midwives and doctors sometimes put weight on the mother's abdomen to aid this process. But usually a few pushes from the mother are enough to help propel the placenta down the birth canal. Out it slithers, bloody and soft, weighing slightly more than a pound. It looks strange if you've never seen one. The placenta is fibrous on the side where it was attached to the uterus and smooth on the baby-facing, amniotic-sac side.

The midwife or doctor will always closely examine the afterbirth (as the placenta is now termed) to be sure it has all come out. Any piece of placenta left behind in the uterus will cause hemorrhage (bleeding).

If for some reason (insufficient contractions, for instance, or extra-strong bond of the placenta to the endometrium) third-stage labor takes too long (more than an hour) and there is some concern about hemorrhage, the accoucheur may try to help stimulate contractions by kneading the woman's abdomen or administering some form of oxytocin. Or the attendant may pull *gently* on the cord. (Vigorous pulling is not recommended, but does occur; it can cause serious bleeding problems.) If these efforts avail nothing, the midwife or doctor may have to extract the placenta manually, a "formidable procedure" in the words of veteran English midwife Maggie Myles.

In most hospitals it is routine to administer to the mother an injection of an oxytocin-type hormone immediately after birth in order to encourage the final uterine contractions. The childbearing process is designed, however, to supply the needed encouragement naturally. That is, if the mother suckles her infant immediately after birth—as more and more mothers in hospitals are nowadays being permitted to do—the newborn's sucking causes certain hormonal secretions which stimulate further uterine contractions, serving to expel the afterbirth and clamp down on the blood vessels of the placental site on the endometrium. This will effectively inhibit the potential for bleeding. In mothers where this process has been interfered with, bleeding is likely to be greater.

The amazing placenta is then thrown away. In some cultures, and often among home birth adherents, the placenta (like the cord) is treated ceremonially. Some people bury it and plant a tree over it as a remembrance of the birth (it would greatly enrich soil!). Some eat it in stew or sautéed—placenta is the only meat that can be eaten without killing a creature. (Constance Bean tried a bite at a Boston area home birth: the flavor was all right in a liver sort of way, she reports in *Labor & Delivery*—but she quietly put down the rest somewhere.)

VARIATIONS AND COMPLICATIONS

One reads the figures repeatedly, and they are on the lips of most midwives, nurse-midwives, childbirth educators, and obstetricians: 90% of births are by nature uncomplicated. For this great majority of people, the preceding description of labor is essentially applicable, with the possible addition of some mild medication or optional procedures (described in Chapter 3).

But statistics are statistics, and perhaps ten times in a hundred, perhaps more often, variations and complications do occur.

During the period of pregnancy most women and men fantasize to some extent about complications and tragedies, about the baby's condition (or survival) and the mother's health as well. This is entirely natural. The class, teacher, or book which overemphasizes problems and emergencies feeds the mother's normal fears and tensions— which is usually counterproductive to the mother's best interests in childbirth preparation. On the other hand, preparation which does not at all deal with these possibilities increases confusion and trauma for those parents who must undergo the unexpected. Here I will describe some of the more statistically likely variations, while urging you to remember that your best contribution to a safe, anxiety-free labor is education and physical preparation, that complications—even tragedies— are easier to deal with if you remain on an even keel and rely upon the preparation and trust you have been developing with those who will be present at your child's birth.

There are many causes, suspected causes, and related phenomena when complications occur. Here are some:

—Aspects of the mother's condition: if she is under 20 or over 35; if she has had more than 5 children (this is called grand multiparity); if she is hypertensive, diabetic, syphilitic, addicted to drugs (such as alcohol or heroin), or malnourished; if she has contracted rubella (German measles) in the first trimester of her pregnancy.
—Oddities in the number or lie of the infant(s) in the uterus or disproportion between the fetus' size and mother's pelvic size.

—Problems which sometimes arise during labor as a result of conditions of the placenta and cord.

—Incompatibility in Rh factor between maternal and fetal blood.

—Labor and birth before the baby is mature enough in all his systems (prematurity) or failure of labor to begin when the appropriate term of uterine life has expired (postmaturity).

—Diseases that strike the mother in late pregnancy (like toxemia and pre-eclampsia) or immediately after birth (sepsis).

This section, exploring some of the factors enumerated above, considers the more common complications that would have to be dealt with at the time of labor. It also describes several conditions which might influence the management of labor and about which the expectant couple ought to be informed. As it turns out, the last two anecdotes in this section—those of Karen and Robin—illustrate how sometimes the efforts of medical intervention, even in problematic situations, serve only to further complicate an already-existing complication.

The Rh factor

Rh is a substance present in the blood of some 86% of us; it coats the red blood cells. People with Rh in their blood are called Rh-positive. The other 14% of us do not have this substance, and are Rh-negative. As a result of the adult body's immunological system, Rh incompatibility between mother and fetus—if not detected early enough in pregnancy—will complicate the management of labor. Either mother or child, or both, may be affected.

Fortunately, the authors of *A Child Is Born* remind us, Rh complications are rare. "There are too many factors that must occur simultaneously for Rh immunity to appear." Yet responsible preparation for childbirth entails an understanding of how the problem may develop and what can be done about it.

When a mother is Rh-negative and the father is also Rh-negative, there is no problem. But if the baby's father is Rh-positive, then there is a chance that the fetus is Rh-positive, and thus different from the mother in whom it is growing. A problem exists when the mother's system develops antibodies to counter the foreign substance. In a first pregnancy this may not be a problem, as the blood transfer during pregnancy is almost all in the direction of mother to child; antibodies would thus not be likely to develop in the mother. At birth, however, with the separation of the placenta from the uterus, some of the baby's blood enters the mother's bloodstream, and her Rh-negative blood produces antibodies to fight the Rh-positive presence. (This could happen during the pregnancy, if the placenta is injured and some fetal blood cells then enter the mother's system.) In a subsequent pregnancy these antibodies would attack the red blood cells of the growing fetus (if that fetus is Rh-positive), causing anemia, massive defects, or fetal death.

The Rh-negative woman produces these antibodies if she has had a miscarriage or an abortion of an Rh-positive child, as well as if she has delivered a living Rh-positive child.

It is only in the last ten years that Rh-negative mothers have had medical relief from the fear of this occurrence. Rh immunoglobulin (trademark RhoGAM), if injected into the mother within 72 hours of delivery, abortion, or miscarriage of an Rh-positive offspring, prevents the mother's immunity system from creating the antibodies. Before this method was developed, one baby in 200 was affected and over half of these died either just before or shortly after birth. Of the others, many were severely impaired.

An Rh-positive newborn whose system contains the life-threatening antibodies must receive a supply of fresh blood in order to survive. A doctor who from prior testing of the mother is aware of an Rh problem will be prepared for an exchange transfusion at the time of birth. To facilitate the procedure, early induction of labor may be the method of choice.

If an Rh-positive fetus is suffering in its uterine life from the attack of the antibodies, medical science can provide it with a blood transfusion *in utero*.

Amniocentesis, usually performed at 14 to 16 weeks of pregnancy, is the procedure whereby a long, hollow needle is inserted through the abdominal and uterine walls in order to withdraw a sampling of fluid from the amniotic sac. A valuable technique for diagnosing the Rh problem *in utero*, amniocentesis has other important diagnostic applications as well (especially for identifying *Down's* syndrome and other chromosomal aberrations).

Fetal distress

This general term describes a condition of the baby before birth when the fetal heartbeat fails significantly to stay within a safe range (110 to 160 beats per minute) because of an insufficiency of oxygen.

Some fetal distress is present in about 25% of births. In about 90% of cases of fetal distress, the cause is compression of the umbilical cord, which may be wrapped around a fetal limb or be pressed between the baby and some part of the mother.

Often the distress is temporary and does not inflict harm. The heartbeat of the fetus naturally varies during labor, as oxygen supply from the mother varies and as the baby is pressed, pushed, and squeezed; it is only when the natural patterns of variations are severely interrupted that distress is present. Various stages of distress include anoxia, hypoxia, bradycardia, brachycardia, asphyxia—conditions all indicating that life-giving oxygen is not getting to the fetus in sufficient amounts.

Presentation

The term presentation (*verb*, to present) refers to the position of the fetus in relation to the neck of the uterus. As labor begins, 95% of babies are presenting head-down in the pelvis, as if to dive forward. This presentation, of the head, is called *vertex* (Latin, ''top'' or ''crown of head''). About 3% of infants present the *breech*, or the rear end (a term from our Anglo-Saxon obstetrical heritage, meaning ''that which would be covered by britches''). Foot-first babies are footling breeches. Of the other 2%, some present face or brow first, and some eschew the longitudinal position altogether and lie cross-wise, a presentation known as *transverse*. Transverse babies cannot be delivered vaginally; either they turn around into a vertex or breech position, or they get born abdominally by Caesarean section.

Another variation includes babies who, though head-down, face the mother's front instead of her back. This *posterior* presentation makes second-stage labor longer and harder for the mother; the pushing must be more strenuous. With a posterior baby, discomfort in the back is constant and considerable. The first stage of labor might also be longer since by nature's design the baby's head, flexed as it is in two-thirds of vertex presentations is the most effective dilator of the cervix.

Danger to the baby in a breech position is considered to be about three times greater than danger in normal vertex presentation. As usual, it is oxygen supply that is at stake; cord compression is not rare. Since the 16th century, doctors have been interested in trying to turn a baby who was in an awkward position; such a procedure is called *version*, and is either external (cephalic) or internal (podalic). External version—trying to turn a baby around to face head-down by manipulating him from the outside, that is, by manipulating the mother's abdomen—can reduce breech presentation from 3% to 2%; the procedure is not without critical hazards, however, such as pulling loose of the placenta. Internal version is almost never attempted, except for removing the second twin; it is a task requiring split-second timing and great manual skill. That's how little Matthew got out.

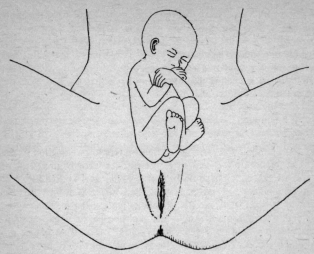

Breech Presentation. This baby is presenting the buttocks first. Three percent of labors involve either this complication or the foot-first variety (footling breech). Labor is harder for mother and baby in such cases.

Harriet carried her fraternal twins, Danny and Matthew, to term; that is, they were born only about 12 days before the due date. Twins are often burdened with prematurity; these boys were not, although the difference in their sizes is quite striking, indicating that Danny had the favored position *in utero*. He came out first, a healthy 6 pounds 1 ounce. Matthew was low-birth-weight for his gestational age, but sturdy at 4 pounds 10 ounces. As usual with multiple births, the obstetrical team was acting conservatively regarding medication. Harriet pushed Danny out after an undrugged and stenuous labor of some 8 hours; his presenting part happened to be arm and neck, so he had some turning to do but finally did slide out.

Then they were telling Harriet to "Push!" It is important to get the subsequent babies out quickly when there is a multiple situation. Risks abound if the fetus stays inside too long—cord prolapse and other oxygen-related concerns, for instance—and twin babies are almost all small or premature in any event. It became clear that Harriet's encore was the one in a hundred who lies transverse. The attendants wanted her to try to nudge him into a longitudinal position so he could be born. But Matthew wasn't budging. So then, Harriet says, they were yelling, "It's stuck! It's stuck!" and then, "Stop pushing!" Whereupon they ordered Harriet's husband out of the delivery room and the gas mask came down on her mouth. The next thing she was conscious of was the first stitch in the unanesthetized suturing up of a generous episiotomy.

In those few minutes that she was out, the doctors had performed a rare and dramatic obstetrical feat: internal podalic version, invented in 1555 by Ambroise Paré in Paris. In this procedure, the accoucheur reaches up through the birth canal, through the dilated cervix and into the uterus; he grasps the foot (or feet) of the transverse fetus and draws it (them) toward and out of the cervix. Footling breech delivery is then accomplished.

In a typical vertex presentation it is the largest part (head) of the fetus that leads the way, the shoulders being next largest, and the trunk the thinnest. Thus when dilation is sufficient for the first part, the rest slips out relatively easily. However, in vaginal delivery of breech babies, it is successively larger parts that are born, each with its own internal rotation. The large after-coming head cannot mold and maneuver around the insufficiently stretched out cervix and birth canal, and fetal hypoxia (oxygen deficiency) can result. In vaginal delivery of breeches, sometimes the cool air of the delivery place shocks the baby's already-born lower parts, and he takes a breath while his mouth is still unborn.

Obstetricians are increasingly turning to Caesarean section to deliver breeches (as high as 50%). If the fetus doesn't voluntarily settle into a more favorable position before labor begins, and cannot be encouraged by external versions to do so, most obstetricians (according to *Williams Obstetrics*) will look hard for an additional reason to justify Caesarean delivery in all but the very immature fetus.

It's a dying art, the art of vaginal delivery of a breech baby. When I spoke recently to my obstetrician he said there hadn't been a vaginal delivery of a breech in ages at the large University-related hospital where he practices. He had done one not so long ago and he said it was like Grand Central Station in there, everyone wanting to observe this rare operation in which the skill and experience of the doctor or midwife weigh heavily on determining the baby's health or survival.

Yet at The Farm, an 1100-person commune in Tennessee, the resident midwives have in recent years delivered 10 breeches at home while taking only 7 to the local hospital for medical consultation and assistance. The experiences of The Farm midwives have shown that breech presentation does not *automatically* dictate medical intervention. A large part of it has to do with the mother's will, support, and state of mind.

Multiple birth

In the U.S., twins occur once in every 93 white births and once in every 78 non-white births. When there is more than one fetus to be delivered, the complications are considerable. Multiple birth is one of the most dramatic and tricky parts of an obstetrician's work; midwives and others rarely manage such a delivery except in an emergency. It is a high-risk situation, capable of changing at the drop of a hat.

Babies who must share nutrition, oxygen, and cramped pelvic quarters are often premature or of low birth weight. One or both may well be in breech position, thus increasing the risk to them. Cord prolapse—the falling down of the umbilical cord (before anything else) into the birth canal—is not uncommon. Multiple pregnancy also predisposes to toxic conditions in the mother. Caesarean section, performed sometimes with twins, is chosen often when there are three or more infants. Yet analgesic and anesthetic medications are particularly dangerous to twins, as to any fetus at risk. The births of Danny and Matthew, described in the preceding section, suggest some of the drama in the delivery room when there's more than one child.

Placenta problems

There are two serious complications of labor which concern the placenta. In both conditions the placenta is not attached where it should be.

Should the placenta come loose from the uterine wall before the baby is safely breathing on its own, a serious threat to the baby's oxygen supply exists. Such abruption of the placenta, or *abruptio placenta*, may announce itself with bright red blood passed vaginally —unless there is a concealed hemorrhaging, which is more serious. Immediate delivery, probably by Caesarean section, is indicated. Recent work indicates that with the right kind of transfusions, delivery may safely follow as long after as 18 hours.

Among the causes of placental abruption are maternal malnutrition, violence of overly stimulated contractions (as in oxytocin-regulated labors), shortness of the umbilical cord, rise in maternal blood pressure, and grand multiparity (a woman who has delivered at least 5 times). The condition occurs once in approximately 100 labors.

Sometimes the placenta grows partly or completely over the cervical opening, obstructing the exit of the fetus and causing bleeding at onset of labor. This serious condition, which occurs once in about 300 deliveries, is called *placenta previa*. Like placental abruption, it is more likely in older women and in women of high parity. The sign of placenta previa is bleeding. As with abruption, the bleeding that heralds the problem is not like the flecks of blood you might see when (if) you pass the cervical mucous plug; it is more considerable, and bright red. Once placenta previa has been diagnosed (by sonography, for instance), delivery is usually brought on forthwith if the fetus is within 3 weeks of maturity. If the condition appears when labor is already under way, Caesarean section is the immediate method of delivery.

Prematurity and postmaturity

If the experience of labor and early neonatal life is a stress for a full-term infant, it is so many times over for a fetus whose system is not ready to sustain itself in extra-uterine life. Much research and writing have been done about the causes and management of prematurity; yet it still remains the reason for more than half the deaths of newborns in the United States. Postmaturity also is a major concern.

Approximately 95% of babies are born between the 266th and the 294th day (38th and 42nd week) of pregnancy—that is, within the ten lunar months plus or minus two weeks. The *premature* infant is the infant born at less than 38 weeks' gestation. The so-called low-birth -weight infant is of any gestational age, but smaller than 2500 grams (5.5 pounds). Low-birth-weight infants face some of the same problems as premature infants.

Generally, the pre-term infant has a body much less fortified to take the stress of labor, to begin digesting colostrum or formula, to obtain oxygen through breathing, and to self-regulate temperature. Premature babies are 30 times more likely to die in early days than full-term infants.

Malnutrition, teenage pregnancy, heavy cigarette smoking, multiple fetuses, alcoholism or drug addiction, maternal hypertension (high blood pressure), diabetes, toxemia, or eclampsia in the mother—these conditions predispose labor to begin too early; consequently the fetus may be retarded in growth. As *Our Bodies, Ourselves* points out, socioeconomic factors may be operative in instances of prematurity. The poor do get less prenatal care, are more inclined to poor nutrition, and deliver many more premature and low-birth-weight infants.

It sticks, too, as a trend; having once given birth prematurely there is a 25% chance of doing so again, and after two the likelihood jumps to 50%.

Premature labor often begins with rupture of the membranes. This makes the uterus and fetus vulnerable to infection. The obstetrical team must then weight the alternatives: (1) to avoid infection, permit labor (i.e., refrain from labor-inhibiting medication), and risk the dangers of prematurity; or (2) to assess that delivery at this gestational age is too risky for the fetus, and allow the last two or three weeks of gestation to occur in as antiseptic an environment as possible. Such compound safety concerns—the calling of high-risk obstetrics—require considerable skill by the obstetrical team in determining the optimal management of the situation.

As with other high-risk situations, premature labor needs to be conducted so as to minimize stress to the fetus. This means avoiding sedatives and narcotics, being even more inclined to do episiotomies, and standing by to resuscitate an infant who may barely be classifiable as living. And so because we can save premature babies we have had to create a branch of medicine to help them reach full health despite the extreme immaturity of most of their systems. The dramatically developing fields of neonatology and perinatology are the specialties which address these problems. Elliott McCleary's *New Miracles of Childbirth* documents the development of this technology.

Among the challenges a premature infant faces, respiration is the first. *Respiratory distress syndrome* (RDS) is the main killer of premature babies and is in fact the major cause of neonatal death in the U.S. Also known as hyaline membrane disease, RDS is characterized by a sticky substance which prevents the infant from being able to breathe successfully. Death comes during the first three days of life. The condition, according to McCleary, affects 5% to 10% of premature babies.

At the other extreme, a baby born more than two weeks late is considered *postmature*. Some 6% to 12% of overdue babies find their uterine world shriveling up on them. If labor has not begun after about the 294th day (42nd week) of pregnancy, the placenta usually begins to shut down, to calcify, and the danger to the fetus is acute. The fetus may have continued to grow past term, and thus be large enough to make labor difficult or prevent vaginal delivery altogether; Caesarean section may be necessary. On the other hand, the fetus may have failed to continue growing during its prolonged uterine residence. Indeed, it may have been starving and losing weight since the end of the "normal" gestation period. Moreover, aspiration of meconium—the fetus breathes in amniotic fluid containing its own defecation (meconium)—carries the danger of pneumonia, and often occurs in postmature babies during the trauma of labor.

The chance of complications, or even stillbirth, is of course greater with postmature than with term babies; whatever the reason for their lateness, their systems are not fully healthy. Unfortunately, inducing labor for the postmature fetus often leads to worse outcomes than leaving such pregnancies alone yet longer.

Toxemia, pre-eclampsia, eclampsia

Toxemia used to be the name given to that threatened state when pregnancy would just seem to get out of control. A woman would retain quantities of water, become bloated, gain much weight, and generally feel very sick. Toxemia and the related conditions pre-eclampsia and eclampsia are very specific disorders of a sort called *hypertensive*. Women already with high blood pressure, diabetes, or kidney disease, women who are in poor health, and women under 16 or over 40 are more likely to be vulnerable. Seven percent of first labors in this country entail some such complication.

From the Greek word meaning "arrow poison," toxemia is a pathologic condition of the mother's blood that may be manifest in late pregnancy by symptoms of pre-eclampsia (and, later, eclampsia): very high blood pressure, swelling of tissues (edema), weight gain, and protein in the urine (proteinuria). Pre-eclampsia may come to a second stage, marked by visual problems, abdominal pain, and headache. If untreated pre-eclampsia progresses to eclampsia, a rare development, characterized by convulsions, often coma, often death of the mother. In at least a third of such cases the baby dies also. The occurrence of convulsions will drastically affect the course of labor and necessitate medical intervention. But prevention, not intervention, is what is most needed; and the toxemic conditions can often be prevented. Nutrition, we shall see, is the key.

Karen is one of the few mothers I know who has experienced a toxemic/eclamptic condition. The experience was so frightful and unexplained, she says, it took her three-and-a-half years to understand what had happened to her, or to feel ready to go through pregnancy, labor, and delivery again. As is usual, however, eclampsia did not recur after the first birth.

Karen, a healthy woman in her early 20s, was eating a good diet, and looking forward to a natural childbirth for her first baby. She began retaining fluid at about five months; during one month she gained 25 pounds from water. As the due date approached, she felt sicker and sicker; she felt "poisoned." On her due date, her doctor noted that Karen was already dilated 4 cm—but he was scheduled to go on vacation. The doctor's stand-in told her to cut out salt (of which she had had none in four months), but generally hesitated to become involved in Karen's case because she was somebody else's patient.

Nearly five weeks later, a full month after her due date, Karen passed bloody discharge. There were no other signs of labor. The stand-in doctor decided she should check in at the hospital and have labor induced the next morning. She was, he declared, pre-eclamptic.

Karen woke up in the hospital at 6:00 A.M. and suddenly experienced a huge contraction. One hour and 20 minutes later Tasha was born.

During that hour and 20 minutes Karen had five *convulsions*, the first one on the litter heading for the labor room. "If this is labor, you can have it" was what she thought of that. Then the fetal heart monitor was hitched up, and then it was decided that indeed Karen really was sick and the baby needed help too.

While Karen was being prepared for Caesarean section with spinal anesthesia, the baby, although posterior, had been inching along. Karen suddenly announced a need to bear down; her baby, to everyone's surprise but her own, was already crowning. They whizzed her down the hall to the delivery room and rolled her onto the table, where she had another convulsion. After much ado, in which she resisted anesthesia and forceps' application, Karen combined one strong push with manual pressure to the top of her uterus and Tasha was born.

When it was all over, the unusual placenta was being passed around with great interest by the obstetrical team.

As it happened, Karen's normally retroverted (tilted back) uterus had straightened up during the first few months of the pregnancy, and in the process had put a kink into the placenta, so that for the last half of pregnancy the fetus was getting limited nourishment. One section of the placenta was dried up, and the cord was thin. This had caused the extra month of pregnancy—the system's effort, in some sense, to provide more time for nourishing, since the amount reaching the fetus had been inadequate.

In Karen's story, the placental problem had been responsible for the lack of fetal nourishment and the eclamptic condition. This might have been diagnosed earlier, but would have been difficult to prevent. Many instances of inadequate fetal nourishment, however, derive from *maternal* malnutrition. Thus, although no one is certain about the reasons for the development of toxemias in pregnancy, two things can be said: (1) toxemia of pregnancy is often a preventable condition; and (2) like prematurity, the distribution of this problem is not random over the population; it hits poor people hardest.

In *Metabolic Toxemia of Late Pregnancy* one Dr. Thomas Brewer reports on his finding of a direct causal relationship between malnutrition in pregnancy and five serious disorders: metabolic toxemia of late pregnancy (toxemia), abruptio placenta, severe newborn and maternal-fetal infection, maternal anemias, and high incidence of low-birth-weight infants. Brewer also sees maternal malnutrition as the cause of many birth defects, including some of the central nervous system.

Brewer began treating toxemia of pregnancy over 20 years ago in rural Louisiana. The rate of incidence there was around 25%. There was also a large number of abruptions, anemias, low-birth-weight infants, infections, and damaged babies. At the time, routine treatment for toxemia included restricting salt, restricting weight gain, and prescribing diuretics (drugs that cause an increase in urination, to cut down the edema, or swelling).

Then Dr. Brewer began treating middle-class women. He noticed that toxemia was practically non-existent. Brewer became convinced that the diuretics rage—drug companies in the late '50s were hard-selling them—was "covering up the real problems of maternal-fetal malnutrition." Further study of the problem began to reveal that the standard medical course of treatment for toxemia was in fact exacerbating the very problem. His solution: good nutrition, especially extra protein. His results at his clinic in Richmond, California: much reduced incidence of low-birth weight and premature infants.

McCleary calls Brewer the Ralph Nader of obstetrics. The ACOG (American College of Obstetricians and Gynecologists) is only beginning to address the issue of education about nutrition, despite the encouraging statistics from Brewer's Richmond clinic. His mothers, if you will, eat better, gain more weight, and bear larger and healthier babies.

Both the frustration experienced by Karen and the motivation of Dr. Brewer share an insight which has been aptly stated in *Our Bodies, Ourselves:* "The emphasis in medicine is almost always placed on making medical intervention more reliable rather than on making medical intervention unnecessary."

Sepsis: past and present

On the whole, the health of the mother is usually sturdier and less in jeopardy than that of the infant. There are, however, three maternal complications which doctors and midwives must always look out for. Hypertension, as in toxemia, is one of them. Hemorrhage from the placental site (described in the section "Third Stage: The After-birth") is another. *Sepsis,* a medical term for infection, is the third.

During the time of pregnancy, labor, and birth, the uterus is extremely vulnerable to infection. This is one reason for the concern a doctor or midwife shows if your waters break and you do not go into labor: a pathway for infection has opened up. Midwives, nurses, and doctors are always very careful about doing internal exams, and, for this reason also, generally try to do as few as possible. Today real danger from sepsis is rare. But even as recently as 130 years ago a birth primer for women would have had to list as one of the worst risks in hospital birth *childbed fever* (also known as puerperal fever, puerperal sepsis, puerperal septicemia), deadly killer of mothers for 200 years.

Epidemics of this scourge would spread through lying-in (maternity) hospitals in Europe and America, killing as many as one mother in four. Before such hospitals existed, the disease was virtually unheard of. But starting in the 17th century it could cost a woman her life to give birth at the hospital. *Except,* on the wards where midwives rather than doctors attended, there was almost no puerperal fever!

Adrienne Rich tells the story of puerperal fever in *Of Woman Born*—how it became a plague; how in the 1850s and 1860s Ignaz Semmelweis in Vienna and Oliver Wendell Holmes in Boston tracked down the disease and found it alive and deadly on the cadaver-bloodied hands of physicians; and how Semmelweis got his fellow doctors to wash with chlorinated lime before attending a puerpera, bringing down the death rate to the level in the midwives' wards. But neither Holmes nor Semmelweis was popular for the discovery. Overwhelmed by feelings of guilt for the deaths he felt he had caused, and discouraged by the general antagonism to his work, Semmelweis on the brink of insanity died from an infection in a wound he had received while operating.

Hospital sepsis is no longer the rule. But a 1965 account of one woman's experience in Boston Lying-In Hospital, Oliver Holmes' own bailiwick, illustrates the continual need for antiseptic care.

Moderately anxious about the prospect of her first childbirth, and anticipating a mild anesthetic, Robin went to the hospital as instructed by her obstetrician to have labor induced. A well-known and very busy doctor, he preferred to induce, and thus ruptured Robin's membranes that morning according to plan. Her labor was managed with Demerol and scopolamine (see Chapter 3), putting Robin into a half-awake, "twilight" state of consciousness. She could hear herself speaking, as if from a distance, and experienced a dreamlike sensation of climbing a wall and having an immovable obstacle between her legs. When labor was just about over late in the afternoon, the doctor then had the standard spinal anesthetic administered. By today's more conservative standards, Robin had been very heavily medicated. At 6 o'clock that evening David was born.

Too blurry from drugs to get involved with her baby, Robin slept. By the next evening she was feeling distinctly sick, showing a 100-degree fever. The fever continued to climb while Robin's abdomen swelled up as if still inhabited by her son; it was intensely sore as well. An obstetrical resident reassured her that it was *not* just postpartum blues.

But what was it?

There were X rays, there were consultations. A tube was put down her throat to pump out the stomach and to relieve swelling. Antibiotics (tetracycline) were given. Twelve hours later, when her fever hit 104 degrees, the obstetrician decided to operate for acute appendicitis. Given the high probability of risk in this procedure (the level of illness was serious already), the obstetrician called in a surgical consultant. Robin, half-delerious, could hear them in grave discussion in the hall outside her room.

Then came an older doctor, who happened to know Robin. He had checked out the case and told the others that this was not appendicitis.

"It's the old enemy," he said. "This is childbed fever. You've never seen it, so you don't know."

So they didn't operate. They gambled on his experience, and they all won: by the next morning the fever had begun to respond to the tetracycline. It *was* puerperal sepsis. Ten days later Robin and her son went home.

Meanwhile, 30 more cases of the fever had broken out in that hospital, a genuine epidemic, and nobody could figure out where the bacteria had come from. After exhaustive detective work it emerged that the anesthesiologist had had two boils on his hand. In taking the pulses of the women to whom he would be giving spinal anesthesia, he passed the bacteria to their hands. The women, following instructions to personally clean the perineum with special soap and little gauze pads, had thereby infected themselves.

POSTPARTUM PERIOD

Immediate

Immediately after birth the activities which focus on the mother include sewing up any tear or cut in the perineum, and examining to see whether bleeding is excessive. The baby is watched for breathing, warmth, and signs of vitality in general. Two routine procedures will then be carried out in any hospital, in most maternity centers, and by most accoucheurs in a home setting: (1) Apgar scoring; (2) eye medication. In a hospital, there will also be footprinting. The last is self-explanatory and is useful for guaranteeing that peoples' babies don't get mixed up—a potential problem only in hospital obstetrical

APGAR SCORING

	Score: 2	Score: 1	Score: 0
Color	Pink	Body pink, limbs bluish	Blue
Pulse	100-plus	Under 100	Zero
Reflex (when soles of feet are slapped)	Cries vigorously	Grimaces	No response
Muscle tone	Moving actively	Moving somewhat	Limp
Breathing	Strong, with strong cry	Slow, irregular, needs help	No respiration

wards, where the baby is often whisked off to the nursery before the parents have had a chance to become acquainted with him or her.

Apgar scoring is a system for rating the overall health of the newborn according to five categories. The neonate is given a rating of either 0, 1, or 2 in each of the five categories; thus the optimal health score is 10. A very pink, very active baby will usually score 9 or 10. A baby who stays bluish, can't get his breathing going strong, and has poor muscle tone would receive a rating around 5.

The scoring is done one minute after birth and again five minutes after birth. The five-minute score is more crucial in estimating the overall health of the new baby.

Virginia Apgar, M.D., Professor of Pediatrics at Cornell University, devised this system in 1953. Her book *Is My Baby All Right?* discusses birth defects authoritatively and with compassion. In most states it is required by law to record an Apgar score for every hospital and nonhospital birth. Parents should have access to these scores.

Eye treatment is also routinely administered. Should the mother be afflicted with gonorrhea, the baby can develop an eye infection in its passage through the birth canal. To prevent infection, hospitals and most birth attendants apply a silver nitrate solution to the infant's eyes immediately after birth. This causes a burning sensation in the newborn's eyes. Many parents, doctors, and midwives now feel that following an uncomplicated birth the application should be postponed at least 45 minutes or so to allow the parents and baby to get to know each other.

Bonding

Once all the bustling has subsided, the period immediately following an uncomplicated birth is a time of quiet alertness and emotional euphoria for parents who are allowed to be together with their new baby. At this time occurs the phenomenon which Marshall Klaus and John Kennell describe in their book *Maternal-Infant Bonding*—the establishment of powerful attachments between mother and baby, father and baby, and between mother and father.

The neonate, studies have shown in recent years, is not a dull, unseeing, unfeeling creature. A film called "The Amazing Newborn," made at Case Western Reserve University (where Klaus and Kennell are professors of pediatrics), shows some of the capabilities and sensitivities of the newborn; the information is quite striking.

Newborns show visual preferences, for instance. They are attracted to visual contrast, to edges, and to curved lines; and they prefer a normal arrangement of facial features rather than a scrambled arrangement of the same features. Further, the film (much slowed down) shows a newborn moving her limbs in time with the rhythms of adult speech, even imitating gestures such as opening the mouth.

What Klaus has discovered, in addition to noting the remarkable responsiveness of the newborn, is that maternal-infant attachment occurs in humans as with other mammals: right after birth, mothers and their offspring form an important bond. The mother must recognize the offspring as hers; then she will protect it. There is a sensitive period after birth when this happens optimally. Bonding is essentially accomplished by sight, touch, and smell. Eye-to-eye contact and skin-to-skin cuddling are the all-important. In *Spiritual Midwifery* The Farm midwives tell how they stay at a birth until the mother has "fallen in love with her baby." Midwife Raven Lang, author of *Birth Book*, likens the process to imprinting in animals.

The study of maternal-infant bonding at Case Western Reserve was first prompted by observing the behaviors of mothers or premature infants. These mothers tended to experience confusion and difficulty in forming a strong attachment with their child after the separation required by the condition of the baby. Research on the possible relationship between maternal-infant separation and subsequent failure of the newborn to thrive is being conducted in England and the U.S.

Klaus recommends that interferences with normal labor and birth be minimized, that conditions favorable to bonding be enhanced. His concern: to look at parturition not as an end, but as a time for establishing the best possible beginning; to understand the role of the birth process in the ontogenic design. "This original mother-infant bond," write Klaus and Kennell, "is the wellspring for all the infant's subsequent attachments and is the formative relationship in the course of which the child develops a sense of himself. Throughout his lifetime the strength and character of this attachment will influence the quality of all future bonds to other individuals."

Hospital stay

If your labor has been uncomplicated and you have had the opportunity to be together, parents and baby, for an hour or so in the delivery room after birth, you will most likely then be separated. The baby will go to the nursery for observation, and the mother will go to her room.

You will notice in the two or three days following birth that your uterus is cramping (contracting) when the baby nurses and/or as a result of hormonal stimulation. These contractions are called afterpains, the attempt of the uterus to regain its normal size. The effort is more difficult, and thus the pains greater, for the multipara.

One sequel to childbirth that sometimes leads to psychiatric help is the phenomenon known as postpartum depression or "baby blues" ("the blue feeling," as Dr. Spock calls it). Most texts and handbooks on birth treat it as a regular, bothersome, temporary, hormonal aftereffect of birthing. Associated with this feeling are fatigue, the sudden sense of new responsibility (especially in new mothers), and the strain of adapting to the new life of the family. Whether you experience this phenomenon mildly, severely, or not at all, the adjustment after birth is aided if your spouse, friends, or relatives can relieve or assist you in housework and care of other children. Finding someone to talk to about the changes you are experiencing, whether that someone is a friend or a counselor, can also be of value.

The incidence of postpartum depression has been observed to be lower in home-birth mothers than in hospital-birth mothers, suggesting that the familiarity and comfort of a home birthing make the transition to motherhood easier.

A standard hospital stay is five days. Many maternity centers and some hospitals allow mothers and babies to leave after three days. Such variables as your own level of fatigue, your need for help from the nursing staff, your tolerance of continual visits from hospital personnel will affect how long you wish to stay. Flexibility of hospital policy and, of course, the medical assessment of your condition and the baby's are the other important determinants.

Hospitals vary in their willingness to allow mother and baby to room together during the hospital stay. Traditionally, after birth the hospital would whisk the newborn off to the nursery and the mother back to her room; baby would be brought to mother for feedings on a fixed schedule and would otherwise be cared for and observed by nurses. Increasingly, however, parents are asking for *rooming-in,* that is, having the baby in the room with the mother either all the time or from early morning until about 9:00 P.M. Rooming-in offers the chance to get to know your baby at your leisure, and, most importantly, to establish feeding with skilled help nearby. Especially if this is your first baby, you may be very glad for help; that first bath can be a shaky affair. Also, with rooming-in the father is able to hold his baby, get acquainted, feel his parenthood.

The puerperium

This term usually describes the time following birth, and designates it as a special period. The time period for the puerperium is usually six weeks. It can help you to establish a good beginning with your new child if you see this period as one in which you have several specific tasks and can expect several specific effects.

By six weeks after birth, the uterus has returned (involuted) to its non-pregnant size; the vaginal discharge from the placental site on the uterine wall has paled from dark red to colorless and then disappeared; and the stitches from episiotomy or from tearing of the perineum have healed. By six weeks the parents have usually been able to establish some kind of fairly regular pattern of sleep and feeding with the infant. And after four weeks or so they can resume having intercourse.

The most significant aspect of the puerperium is the establishment of feeding in the infant. The choice of breast or bottle is one you will probably have made some time in advance. One benefit of the bottle is that anyone can feed the baby—the father, the baby's siblings, grandmothers, and assorted doting friends. In my mother's time (early 1940s), one was a genuine oddity if she intended to breastfeed. The pro-medication attitude of the 40s and 50s included at best neutrality toward nursing. Most people at the time suggested that it was neater, more scientific, and more liberated to use formula. Some of us now sustain allergies, eczema, bronchitis, hay fever, and colds as a result of this cultural attitude.

Finally breastfeeding is coming back. La Leche League International (see Chapter 6) is the organization which has for twenty years devoted itself to promoting breastfeeding and helping mothers gain success at it. Their book *The Womanly Art of Breastfeeding* is a classic. Indeed, breastfeeding is the subject of many books and countless articles. The case in favor of it is continually being supported by research findings.

Klaus and others point out from empirical evidence that breastfed babies have fewer digestive, respiratory, and skin problems and seven times fewer allergies. The really quite indescribable tranquility and warmth and pleasure of nursing a baby is another factor. Bodily contact, the kind of closeness that any holding and feeding operation offers, is the language of the child in its early months. Colostrum is the substance a nursing baby receives from his mother's breast in the three or so days following birth before the milk comes in. It is a substance rich in protein, minerals, various vitamins, and antibodies.

The chance for close contact between father and child is not lost, however, when the mother chooses breastfeeding. The father can still establish a close physical relationship even if in the early months this does not include actual feeding.

Breastfeeding is as sensitive to emotional climate as is lovemaking. If there is strife and worry, the mother and baby, like love partners, have a much harder time relaxing with their relationship. Anxiety, fatigue, and excessively critical attitudes can undo the pleasure of the interaction. "The survival of the race for the millions of years before the concepts of 'conscience' and 'duty' were invented," writes Marshall Klaus, "depended on the intense satisfaction gained from the acts of reproduction. Breastfeeding, like coitus, had to be pleasurable and satisfying if the race were to continue."

Like bonding, breastfeeding is best accomplished in a rooming-in situation. Nursing requires that mother and child be together, learning to be comfortable, responding to signals, learning to relax and to enjoy the feeding. This can be difficult if the hospital nursery is determining the feeding times and "supplementing" the baby's feedings with sugar water, which can undermine the establishment of breastfeeding. If your wish is to nurse your baby, it is important to be supported by the personnel of the facility where you will be spending the intial post-partum days.

Times *have* changed: less than two decades ago a mother wishing to breastfeed her baby would likely have been discouraged by most hospital staffs. Now we are likely to find that, even in a hospital facility which is busy and understaffed, there are nurses who actively support breastfeeding and who offer encouragement and good, practical counsel in a midwifelike way.

2

Ideas of
Natural Childbirth

The Romans named the pain of childbirth *poena magna*, "great pain"; as Adrienne Rich points out, *poena* carries a second meaning: penalty. This is our culture's heritage. In sorrow, says the Bible, thou shalt bring forth children. So goes the story. Woman must suffer in giving birth as God's punishment on Eve for tempting Adam.

And so, in this view, attempts to control or eradicate the pangs of birth were at first regarded as heretical.

In Western culture today, the practice of natural childbirth is founded upon ways of thinking that embrace scientific method, sound psychology, compassion, and common sense. If any form of heresy may yet be said to linger, it would have to be attributed to the often unnecessary interferences to obstetric technology with the natural course of the birth-giving process. In *Pregnancy, Birth & the Newborn Baby*, Margaret Mead offers this observation: "It should be pointed out that natural childbirth, the very inappropriate name for forms of delivery in which women undergo extensive training so that they can cooperate consciously with the delivery of the child, is a male invention, meant to counteract practices of complete anesthesia, which were also male inventions. Contemporary forms of natural childbirth are an attempt to restore to women what women among many peoples once had."

For some of us the term natural childbirth calls forth the image of a strong, primitive woman who stoically labors at some comfortable spot, assisted by wise female relatives and a designated midwife. Unsurprised and unprotesting, she delivers her child. After the appropriate ceremony, she swaddles the infant and resumes her regular routine. There are no issues, no controversies, no alternative methods. There is only the way her people have always done this. The infant remains close to the mother for months following birth, tied to her back or her front as she goes about her normal work in the field, home, garden, wherever. The movements of the mother's body, the ever-available breast, all extend the comfort and security of intra-uterine life and permit a kind, gradual entry into the outer world. Care begins to come quite naturally from other members of the family.

Older children, especially girls, unquestioningly accept the role of little parent, and the elderly often assume the duties of child-watching. In this way the baby is perpetually in the arms of her family, her people, her culture.

We have no such tradition; our experience of labor and delivery is conditioned rather to a wide range of expectations. We are at this time, the late-1970s, learning to sort through the vast collection of techniques and theories concerning childbirth management, to select what works medically and physically and emotionally for us, with our own baggage of fears, conditionings, thresholds, and needs.

In this endeavor we find the term natural childbirth applied with considerable variation. For many, the term is essentially a misnomer, since there is nothing "natural" about the de-conditioning and re-learning processes that are necessary to achieve the method. Educators are as eager to tell us what natural childbirth is *not* as they are to propose what it is. For some it only means childbirth in which there has been no interference whatever from drugs or medical procedures. Suzanne Arms, author of *Immaculate Deception,* writes: "Natural childbirth is not an aggressive action against the forces of nature. Nor is it a suppression of the sensation and experience of the tremendous effort of the body to give birth. It is simply the full experience of the normal sequence of events flowing without interruption from any external disturbances or interference."

But a young woman who has returned from the hospital with her healthy baby, whose birth she saw—even through her head was slightly groggy at the time from a small dose of pain reliever and her birth canal was numb from an epidural anesthetic—she may well feel that she had "natural" childbirth: after all, she was the one who decided to take medication, she arranged the details herself, she was awake and aware as she pushed her child into the world, husband by her side.

Yet the insistence on noninterference as a criterion of natural childbirth reflects the opportunity our society has had in the 1950s and '60s to observe labor in its "natural" state, that is, in a form it had before it began to be habitually interfered with. We are starting to know the birth process, as we are learning what bread is like when it is made from unrefined flour.

Mehitabel, a first-time mother with no instruction whatever, went into labor around midnight one day last spring. At first she showed confusion and restlessness, but with some encouragement settled down and started quite spontaneously to initiate each contraction with a "cleansing" breath. As expulsion approached, she began a shallow, panting rhythm of breathing. All five kittens and afterbirths arrived with minimal trouble, and no drugs were used.

It turns out that when labor is respected it shows us how to deal with it. I visited with a Lamaze-trained woman who stayed in control through the building of contractions as transition approached. In the middle of a contraction she abruptly commenced light, fast breathing, and when the contraction was over she noted that she would be needing that kind of breathing from then on. She had of course known that such a changeover time would come, but the point is that she herself had not *consciously* intiated the shift in breathing. She was staying as relaxed as she could; the contraction itself had told her how to breathe.

Childbirth pain is the pain of the contracting uterus, the muscle swelling, and the pulling open of the cervix. In early labor, this is often felt as an ache in the groin, perhaps low in the back, moving around. Discomfort is perhaps a better word for early contractions. Active labor is a more distinct discomfort. And the pain of the relatively brief transition phase is characterized by an overwhelming, helpless sensation. After transition, the second-stage labor pushing contractions, though strenuous work, are by most women generally not characterized as painful. Stretching open of the vulva is felt as a burning sensation. In her autobiography *Blackberry Winter*, Margaret Mead reflects upon the character of childbirth pain from her own experience of labor in 1939: "All night I felt as if I were getting an attack of maleria, but I did not know—one of those things one does not know—whether the sensation of having a baby might not feel like maleria. And I was fascinated to discover that far from being 'ten times worse than the worst pain you have ever had' (as our childless woman doctor had told us in college) or 'worse than the worst cramps you ever had, but at least you get something out of it' (as my mother had said), the pains of childbirth were altogether different from the enveloping effects of other kinds of pain. These were pains one could follow with one's mind; they were like a fine electric needle outlining one's pelvis."

As recently as 1940 contractions were called pains. This terminology, one must admit, predisposes to discomfort in a way that *contractions* does not. A contraction draws muscle tissue together. A pain hurts.

This change in vocabulary is one prerequisite to any level of achievement of natural childbirth in our society.

Concomitant with the linguistic change is the attitude that childbirth can be something besides a torture, a necessary horror. In this chapter we will consider how doctors, educators, mothers, and fathers have developed philosophies and programs and techniques for dealing *consciously* with the birth experience, regarding it in new contexts, giving it new significances. From this emerges the idea of a course of preparation for childbearing. The basic outline of preparation as most teachers see it will be clear as we look at some of the history of this movement, calling it by its original name, Dick-Read's name for it, natural childbirth.

DR. DICK-READ, DR. LAMAZE,
AND DR. LEBOYER

During the past several decades three European obstetricians have contributed major theories about childbirth and have developed specific techniques related to their ideas. They are Dr. Grantly Dick-Read, Dr. Fernand Lamaze, and, most recently, Dr. Frederick Leboyer. The idea of natural childbirth as it has been developing in Europe and North America for the last thirty years had its conception and early growth in the work of the English obstetrician Grantly Dick-Read.

"It didn't hurt. It wasn't meant to, was it, Doctor?"

When Dr. Dick-Read was practicing obstetrics in London some fifty years ago, a patient of his made a remark which, he says, strongly impressed him and indeed altered the course of his life. It has altered the course of modern obstetrical practice as well.

The patient was a poor woman; Dr. Dick-Read arrived at her home in the middle of the night on his bicycle. Labor progressed normally. The woman politely refused Dr. Dick-Read's offer of chloroform. When Dr. Dick-Read later asked her why, she turned to him and said: "It didn't hurt. It wasn't meant to, was it, Doctor?"

With that, Dr. Dick-Read began reflecting on the incidence of pain in childbirth. Many women, both in Britain and in other lands, such as Africa, where Dr. Dick-Read had practiced, seemed to suffer horribly in giving birth; others, he noted, experienced little pain. What distinguished the relatively painless labors, he came to realize, was a calm, knowing acceptance of the course of labor as normal and natural.

In Dr. Dick-Read's view, it has been culture, civilization itself, which has introduced anxiety and fear into women's expectations regarding birth. Legend and literature of course abound with stories of the agonies suffered by women in labor. And they are as much a part of the culture of more primitive peoples as of ours, these legends of great punishing pain in childbirth.

Let us be clear: the pain is real enough. Though some 7% of women report that they feel none, for most of us it is no fantasy, no imagination. Dick-Read, like many others, realized that this is a pain which can be grasped, altered, transformed, by-passed, reduced.

Fear and the expectation of pain, pondered Dr. Dick-Read, create protective tension in the body, and that tension increases and emphasizes the pain response. Indeed, in a laboring woman, tension fights the uterus in its effort to open up the cervix. This process he calls the Fear-Tension-Pain Syndrome. He concludes that relieving fear, relaxing tension, and thus minimizing pain should be the work of the obstetrician.

Giving birth under such conditions would be closer to the process as designed by nature. His term "natural childbirth" thus means childbirth in which "no physical, chemical or psychological condition is likely to disturb the normal sequence of events or disrupt the natural phenomena of parturition."

Dick-Read emphasizes the spirituality of birth. His admiration for the process gives a warmth to his writing, which may seem old-fashioned, at times even mystical; but it is his caring thoughtfulness that is communicated most clearly.

His first writing on the subject, from 1919, when Dr. Dick-Read was a resident, was based on a dozen years of observing childbirth. By 1929 Dick-Read had collected further evidence, and in 1932 his book *Natural Childbirth* was published in England. Its reception was modest. His major work, *Childbirth Without Fear,* appeared 12 years later, by which time Dick-Read's work was beginning to be known. It is now in its fourth edition and has been translated into a dozen languages. Social acceptance was slow, for Dick-Read's theories so clearly opposed the fashionable trend of the time, namely, grateful acceptance of general anesthesia in labor and delivery to obliterate sensation entirely, and so to liberate the woman from what was considered hideous and unnatural. Dick-Read believed, however, that his theory and the practical advice that went with it would be justifiably triumphant.

This kindly obstetrician had become a crusader. His goal: the right of mothers: "Every woman we attend should be enabled to appreciate the personal triumph of motherhood." The elation and spiritual joy Dr. Dick-Read observed in mothers who were able to deliver consciously, with their own active participation, convinced him repeatedly that this is the way nature intends for birth to occur, that the psychological and physical benefits for the new life and for the family unit are enormous.

Dr. Dick-Read's program proposes four overall conditions for successful childbirth: (1) all young people should be educated about the course of pregnancy and labor to help recondition the entire species to expect strenuous but largely painless childbirth; (2) pregnant women need to be educated about the physiological process they are going through in order to build confidence; (3) attendants in the labor ward must be trained, to be a "bulwark against the onslaught of fear and a tower of strength in time of doubt, weakness, or wavering self-control"; and (4) the doctor must keep in mind the Fear-Tension-Pain Syndrome.

In practical terms, Dr. Dick-Read offers a program of education, breathing, relaxation, and physical fitness. These aspects of his theory are available now as a separate manual, called *The Practice of Natural Childbirth*, published in paperback in 1976.

In this work he presents first his brief version of the physiology of pregnancy in order to prevent anxiety due to ignorance of the physical facts.

Dr. Dick-Read introduces the short section on breathing by pointing out that proper breathing is important to good health in general and essential to the pregnant woman. It is her breathing which, through the placenta, supplies the fetus with its oxygen. During labor, correct breathing is an indispensable aid to the woman who has decided to be conscious and to contribute actively to the birthing.

According to Dick-Read, body relaxation like careful breathing has its role during pregnancy and during all stages of labor, as well as being part of the foundation of good physical and mental health in general. It releases tension, promotes calm and confidence, and of course permits the important circular muscles at the cervix end of the uterus to remain noninterfering. All uterine muscular activity (or nonactivity) can be better understood and accepted in the relaxed, calm, prepared mind.

Relaxation, like breathing control, needs to be practiced by the pregnant woman. Dick-Read instructs the woman to prepare for relaxtion first by setting up the proper conditions: darkened room, emptied bladder, removed dentures; the surfaces should be firm, the knees and head supported slightly. He then describes what instructions he gives in person to the woman learning relaxation.

The relaxed state which Dr. Dick-Read induces is, he says, day-dreamlike; it resembles, of course, the relaxed, aware, deeply replenishing condition offered by various meditation techniques, which are now becoming popular in our society. "Perhaps I may add," he

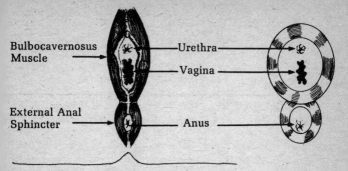

Muscles of the Perineum. This drawing shows the major perineal muscles in their figure-eight arrangement. Learning to tighten and release these muscles is of great value to women, not only during labor.

suggests in *The Practice of Natural Childbirth*, "that the obstetrician himself would be very well advised to become adept at relaxation. Not only would he be more competent to teach his patients or train instructresses, but he would find himself retaining his energy during those long hours of waiting. His mental acuity and manual dexterity would be more efficient also, than if he had remained tense with anticipation during his attendance at the labor."

Dr. Dick-Read offers standard physical exercises. The most important is Firming the Pelvic Floor Muscles, an exercise found in almost every discussion of preparation for childbirth, or postpartum reconditioning. Another name is the Kegel exercise, named for Arnold Kegel, a California physician. The benefits of this particular exercise are not restricted to pregnant women. It consists quite simply of contracting the sphincters (muscles which surround and enclose an orifice) of the anus, of the vagina, and of the urethra even. Regular practice will keep vaginal muscle toned up, thus preventing sagging of the uterus. Obviously this exercise can be done any time, any place; it is suggested that every woman of every age and condition remember to tone up these sphincters by contracting and releasing them many times every day (on the subway, at work, while cooking, while making love). For delivery, control over these muscles is vital. Being able to release them can make it possible to let the baby out gently and with little pain. If these muscles are held tight, tearing and bursting will result at the moment of birth. Leakage of urine is less likely during pregnancy if you have this control, as are hemorrhoids. Furthermore, the stretched vagina will more quickly revert to its

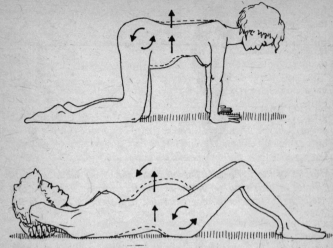

The Pelvic Rock, or Pelvic Tilt. This basic exercise can be done in either of the two positions. The idea is alternately to arch, then flatten, the small of the back; this relieves lower backache.

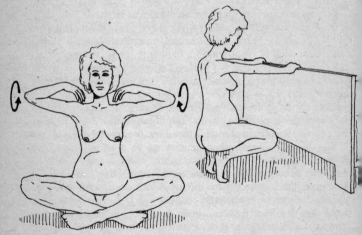

Tailor-Sitting and Squatting. Two basic positions to prepare for maximum stretching of the birth area. Shoulder rotation relieves upper backache.

former tightness after birth if the woman has learned control over these sphincters.

The other exercises include (1) The Pelvic Rock, also an old favorite, to loosen the lower back and relieve backache; (2) Squatting, to stretch the inner thighs and loosen the knees and hips—a practice in "the best position for delivery of the child" (most agree), with variations such as sitting tailor-style (also called "Indian style"); (3) Firming the Breasts, to improve the circulation near the breasts and give breath-holding practice; and (4) Labor Position, to get used to the position which, Dick-Read says, is the most comfortable for giving birth, although it should be noted here that in American hospitals the flat-on-your-back position is most often used. The details on these exercises are succinctly described in Dick-Read's *The Practice of Natural Childbirth*.

His unshakable belief in the value of naturally conducted childbirth does not, as some critics imagine, cause him to oppose the use of anesthetic agents where they are needed or wanted. His contention is rather that 95% of labors are normal, and that with preparation the laboring woman will not wish to be drugged. Over and over again, he is clear: "No woman should be allowed to suffer greater discomfort in labor than she is willing to endure for her child's sake"; and, "When women are in labor there should always be an anesthetic or analgesic apparatus at hand, and if necessary they should be instructed in its use." Dick-Read estimates from his experience that approximately 1% to 3% of mothers giving birth with no complications and prepared in the natural childbirth method will elect to use a form of medical pain relief.

Dick-Read lists his objections to the "anesthesia-for-all" idea, objections which to this day recur frequently in the literature on childbirth, as they are based on varying kinds and amounts of data. They can be summarized as follows:

1. No anesthetic is free of danger to mother and/or child.
2. Anesthesia converts a normal physiological process into a pathological state with the attendant risks.
3. Anesthesia tends to bring with it an increase in use of other interferences, such as forceps, with their risks.
4. Anesthesia interferes with certain occurrences of a natural labor upon which maternal and infant safety depend.
5. Childbirth with anesthesia renders surgical an experience of great spiritual significance.
6. Childbirth without anesthesia enchances the growth of the mother-child bond in a way that is unknown to the mother unconscious of her baby's arrival.

Psychoprophylaxis/the Lamaze method

The best known and most widely practiced systematic approach to childbirth without pain or drugs is the Lamaze method, developed by Fernand Lamaze, an obstetrician from Paris, after he visited the Soviet Union in 1951. While there, at an international conference on childbirth, Lamaze heard about the Soviet method *psychoprophylaxis*, a term meaning prevention of pain by psychological means. The concept is based on the work of Soviet scientists, most notably Ivan Pavlov. At a clinic in Leningrad Lamaze observed the method in use; he was so deeply impressed that upon his return to France he immediately began training personnel in the use of it. His clinic, the Maternité du Metallurgiste, the maternity hospital of the metallurgists' union, became the testing ground for Lamaze's version of the Soviet technique. Lamaze's book, *Painless Childbirth*, was first published in 1958; by that time the Ministry of Health of the Soviet Union had decreed the general application of the method in that country, and the Pope had, in 1956, given the Lamaze technique his official blessing.

How had this method originated? Early in the twentieth century the Soviet scientist Ivan Pavlov conducted his now-famous experiments about conditioned behavior. His subject was a dog. Pavlov would ring a buzzer and then offer food to the dog. After a few dozen trials of this sort, he rang the buzzer but offered no food. The dogs salivated. The dog had been conditioned to salivate to the sound of the buzzer.

In a more complicated version, a dog was simultaneously shocked and fed; Pavlov performed many trials. At first, the dog would whimper and jerk away, uncomfortable and anxious from the shock. After a few days of this, the discomfort/defense reflex diminished, and soon the only response to the shock was salivation. A painful stimulus had been *transformed* by the brain of the dog into a stimulus causing only the salivation reflex.

Pavlovian technique was then applied to pain, and to the pain of childbirth in particular. Thus, in the psychoprophylaxis method, the laboring woman responds to uterine contractions with specific breathing techniques which she has learned and practiced; this focuses her concentration in a way that does not permit the sensation of pain to register. At the same time, of course, it trains the woman for proper breathing during labor.

Lamaze preparation for childbirth is a precise and rigorous system. Beginning in the seventh month of pregnancy the woman is educated and trained. Optimally, a class would be geared to from three to five couples, though enrollment may be much higher. And though the actual classes usually number only six, extensive regular practice at home is necessary to the success of the method. The husband is an indispensable part of the training as exercise coach, timer of contractions, and major support. (The original French version used the services of a trained *monitrice,* or teacher, as coach; the method has been revised to turn this function over to the father.)

The training which Dr. Lamaze instituted a quarter of a century ago is still taught much in the same way today. In the U.S. and Canada, however, the dissemination and popularity of the Lamaze method owe more to the teachings and writings of other individuals than directly to the work of the founder himself. In 1960 Elisabeth Bing, a physical therapist and most ardent disciple of Lamaze, co-founded the American Society of Psychoprophylaxis in Obstetrics (ASPO) in New York. Helping her in this was an American woman, Marjorie Karmel, who delivered her first child in Paris under the care of Dr. Lamaze. Ms. Karmel returned to the U.S. and tried to approximate that experience when her second child was due; the difficulties and adventures she then struggled through led her to write her pleasant, informative, personal account, *Thank You, Dr. Lamaze,* and then to team up with Ms. Bing. Since the founding of the ASPO, the number of Lamaze-trained couples in both North America and Europe is ever on the rise.

The Lamaze training program appears in straightforward form in Ms. Bing's book *Six Practical Lessons for an Easier Childbirth.* Another quite similar version occurs under the title "Manual of Information and Practical Exercises for Painless Childbirth" as an appendix to Ms. Karmel's book. Dr. Lamaze's own book, *Painless Childbirth,* concerns itself primarily with scientific background from the Soviet work of the early twentieth century. Included also is a rendering of his lectures, which are more stiff, clinical, and less accessible than the versions offered by Ms. Bing and Ms. Karmel.

Other books deserve mention at this point, as works whose major premises extend or amplify the pioneering work of both Lamaze and Dick-Read. *Childbirth with Confidence,* by Dr. Pierre Vellay, a colleague of Dr. Lamaze in Paris, includes a description of sexual development from birth through puberty as well as a description of psychoprophylactic method. Some possibly questionable attitudes expressed by Dr. Vellay include his referring to the laboring woman as a schoolgirl who, according to the metaphor, has learned her lessons well, or badly, and his naming the vagina a "slit" for the benefit of children who are at the stage where they insist on asking "the most embarrassing questions." *Childbirth with Confidence* is, however, a technically precise book, and its presentation of the Lamaze method is clear.

Dr. Irwin Chabon's enthusiastic book *Awake and Aware: Participation in Childbirth through Psychoprophylaxis* is another popular interpre-

tation of the Lamaze method, and *Preparation for Childbirth* by
Donna Ewy and Roger Ewy offers a concise guide for the training
parents.

Lamaze, like Dick-Read, stresses the importance of factual education in childbirth preparation. Hence, the Lamaze training program
begins with a moment-to-moment review of the physical processes of
pregnancy and labor. Such preparation serves not only to allay fears
due to ignorance, but also to begin to decondition the parents-to-be.
Conditioning, a key word in the literature of psychoprophylaxis,
refers to learned behavior, certain aspects of which it is the goal of
Lamaze training to alter. Once the factual education is complete and
fearful expectations are alleviated, relearning can begin. Our culture,
claims the Lamaze system, has conditioned us all to expect pain in
childbirth. We must unlearn this expectation and recondition ourselves, replacing old behavior with new, in order to achieve painless
childbirth. The new learning process, whereby a particular stimulus is
connected with a particular response, occurs at the level of impulses
sent to the brain. Lamaze says it like this: "One of the objects of the
method is to enlighten the woman by instructing her about the
phenomena involved in childbirth, the purpose being to convert delivery from the idea of pain to a series of understood processes in which
uterine contraction is the leading phenomenon."

The essential process, then, is to form new conditioned reflexes.
Lamaze reasons that if uterine contractions are associated with strong
enough other stimuli, a conditioned reflex connecting the two could
come into being. Hence the sense of "apprenticeship" which the
expectant mother is to undergo. If one can learn to swim, one can
learn to give birth painlessly. It is verbal instructions, words spoken
by the labor coach (usually the husband), which cue the new
response.

The Lamaze instructor uses exercises to teach a precise set of
breathing techniques appropriate to the various stages of labor. These
new responses, specific breathing techniques, are physiologically
useful as well, providing the correct amount of oxygen to the laboring
body.

The physical exercises are useful in two ways; they limber up the
muscles of the body, aiding in circulation and in general elasticity,
and they begin the training of the woman in specific selected muscle
control. Labor is most efficient when muscular activity and muscular
relaxation are consciously controlled. Uterine contractions represent
involuntary muscular activity; to allow maximal body energy for this
activity, the laboring woman must relax those muscles over which she
does have control. The relaxation compensates for the additional
oxygen supply needed by the hard-working muscles. As an exercise,

learning upon command to relax all muscles *except*, for example, those of the right arm and left leg, will be helpful during labor when such precise control is called for. This would apply, for example, to the expulsive stage of labor, when the pelvic floor muscles (voluntary) must be relaxed while the uterus (involuntary) and the abdomen contract strenuously. It takes practice to become aware of which muscles are working and which are at rest.

The simple specific exercises also begin to teach overall relaxation and the refreshing, deep breath known to Lamaze technique as the *cleansing breath*. The cleansing breath, in which exhalation is deep and full and complete relaxation of the body follows, is practiced at the beginning and end of each exercise; it is the husband (or other coach) who checks the level of relaxation. *Daily* practice of the exercises is recommended. In this way, muscle control can become automatic and close teamwork between wife and husband is established.

The body-building exercises are similar to those of other systems of preparation. Sitting tailor-fashion ("Indian-fashion"), simple leg raising, and raising of the back off the floor with the knees bent from a lying-down position are among those recommended. These exercises are described and demonstrated with photographs in Elisabeth Bing's book, *Six Practical Lessons for an Easier Childbirth*.

The review of physiology, the muscular control exercises, and the general body-building exercises are covered in Ms. Bing's first two lessons. Beginning with lesson three, the specific breathing techniques for use in labor are taught. These breathing techniques are the core of the Lamaze teaching.

The insistence on special breathing, deliberately different from normal breathing, has two aims. First, keeping the breath up in the chest has the previously mentioned purpose of keeping the pressure off the uterus; second, as Ms. Bing explains, in Lamaze technique the aim is to create a strong center of concentration, to train the laboring woman to react to a uterine contraction with a respiratory response instead of a fear/flight response. It makes good sense that the more precise the instructions, the more concentration will be used in the carrying out of them.

Another Lamaze technique which combines a useful physical purpose with an attention-diverting one is taught by Ms. Bing under the heading of "What To Do With You Hands." It is not recommended that one dig her nails into her husband's arm. Instead, suggests the Lamaze method, practice *effleurage*—light, circular massage of the lower abdomen. The technique is described with characteristic precision: inhale as your fingers move up and exhale as they move down, using some talcum powder over the abdomen to prevent skin irritation. Effleurage relieves tension while providing another point of concentration.

The importance of the husband in this training is once again emphasized. He checks the level of your relaxation during practice; and, once contractions begin for real, it is his voice which will be your cue for the automatic responses you have been learning. Thus he is taught to mention that the contraction has begun, to count off its duration ("15 seconds, 30 seconds," etc.), and to note the end of the contraction, the signal for the cleansing breath. (Although the Lamaze technique as it is taught never mentions the possibility that the companion and coach would be anyone but a husband, obviously it could be. A woman I know went through Lamaze training classes and labor with a close female friend as her companion/coach.)

During early first-stage labor, the chest breathing relieves discomfort usually until the cervix is about 3 cm dilated, or almost one-third of its eventual opening up. Then begins the second part of first-stage labor, active (or "accelerated") labor, for which a new method of breathing is taught. At this point contractions usually last 45 to 60 seconds and occur 4 to 5 minutes apart; early-phase breathing is no longer effective in controlling discomfort. Contractions have speeded up; breathing is to be speeded up.

One of the sources of imagery in the Lamaze method is that of races and athletic contests. This may seem unlikely to anyone who has not been in labor, but many find this sort of metaphor appropriate. Labor is enormously intense physical work; fitness and the ability to relax and to use one's body with efficiency do pay off. Another recurrent motif in Lamaze description (and universally, in fact) is that of a wave. A contraction, after all, has a wavelike shape: it begins gradually, builds in intensity and strength to a peak, then decreases and disappears. Women always refer to the need to "get on top of" a contraction; this is like riding on the crest of an ocean wave. The alternative is to allow the wave to get on top of you, to be drowned in it, to have no control.

So, for this middle section of the first part of the race, an accelerated breathing is taught. The uterus has speeded up, and thus needs more oxygen. As a contraction begins, you begin with a cleansing breath and then proceed immediately into *panting*—rapid, short breaths which you speed up as the contraction builds. As the contraction declines, your breathing decelerates and you end with a cleansing breath.

When your cervix is dilated about four fingers' worth, or 8 cm, you are entering transition, the last part of first-stage labor (and the toughest). It is relatively brief, usually 30 to 90 minutes, after which you will have the relief of being able to push.

Transition breathing is the most exacting of the techniques. To stay in control during this time, you will learn a set rhythm of panting breathing followed by *blowing out*. You begin with a cleansing breath at the beginning of the contraction; immediately you are to start panting, since these transition contractions wait for nothing, but build to great intensity at once. Panting is to be done in a rhyhm of four to six pants followed by a blowing out, than panting again, blowing out, until the contraction is over; you end, of course, with a cleansing breath. Lamaze's technique is ready with a remedy should the premature urge to push come to you: blow out. Since pushing is most effectively done with the breath held (think of a bowel movement), it makes sense that one is unable to push while forcibly exhaling.

Panting makes you thirsty, reminds Ms. Bing; perhaps you will be allowed some crushed ice. (A candy stick or a lollipop is also recommended.) At this stage you can also benefit from visual focusing, another little detail in the methodical Lamaze effort. Bring to your birthing place a bright piece of cloth, or a picture you particularly like, pin it on the wall opposite you, and stare at it as you concentrate. Visual focusing, taught by most childbirth instructors, helps to keep your mind centered on the all-important task you are in the midst of.

Once you are 10 cm dilated you begin the second, expulsive stage of labor, which will culminate in the birth of your baby. Breathing strategy for this stage is different from what has occupied you up until this point.

The contractions themselves are not so violent as during transition. Usually there is longer time between them, which you will be glad to use for resting. The most efficient pushing is done after the contraction has reached its peak. Ms. Bing recommends that you take a cleansing breath as one of these contractions begins, then take a second cleansing breath and let it out also, and then take a third and hold it. If you can lift your upper body to an angle of about 45 degrees, all the better; if your husband can help you lift your legs up, as you have been taught in class, this will also aid your efforts. Then you push. You push most and first with the diaphragm, and you are encouraged by Ms. Bing: "Remember! Think in the direction you are pushing." You push for as long as you can, perhaps some 15 seconds, then you let the air out, take another deep breath, and continue, until the contraction is over, at which time you take several deep cleansing breaths to replace the oxygen you have so strenuously been using up.

An absolute essential to the success of this pushing is keeping the pelvic floor relaxed. This is the difference between pushing in expulsive labor and pushing in bowel movement; the perineum in delivery must be as relaxed as is possible, so as not to constrict the passageway through which the baby is moving. If you have practiced your muscular control exercises diligently enor gh, this simultaneously pushing from above and relaxing below will be possible for you.

And, as throughout labor, the voice of your coach telling you to breathe, to blow out, to push, to take another breath, and encouraging this mighty work will add immeasurably to your confidence and ability.

There is one break in all this exertion. As the baby is about to emerge you will be told suddenly to stop pushing. That is to give the vaginal opening a chance to fully stretch to accommodate the infant's head. Pushing while the head is against the perineum may cause a tear. On command, you will lie back and pant, in relaxation, until the urge to push has receded. Then you will push, gently, and your baby will be born.

One may wonder what such a systematic, scientifically-based method has to do with the idea of *natural* childbirth. Indeed, Dr. Lamaze's most ardent disciple, Elisabeth Bing, contends that "the psychoprophylactic method of childbirth . . . is *not* a technique of so-called 'natural childbirth.' On the contrary, it is a technique which is not at all natural, but acquired through concentrated effort and hard work on the part of the expectant mother and her husband. It is a method which provides an analgesic (or lessening of pain) achieved by physical means instead of by drugs or chemical means." Perhaps *prepared* or *educated* childbirth are more accurate terms of describing muc' of what popularly gets labeled as natural. But what psycho-prophylaxis and any idea of natural childbirth share in common is an attitude largely of self-reliance. "Natural childbirth," writes Suzanne Arms, "requires a calm and abiding faith and constant emotional support for a woman to participate in her body as it births itself." So does psychoprophylaxis.

The two major figures in the history of natural or painless or prepared childbirth, Dr. Dick-Read and Dr. Lamaze, have of course been criticized. Dick-Read is considered overly mystical, too religiously inclined, not active enough in preparation. Dr. Lamaze points out that although Dick-Read discovered the importance of relaxation and of education in preparing women for parturition, he cannot have been successful because he knew nothing of conditioned reflexes. Dick-Read for his part, does not mention Lamaze by name, but speaks of "certain French obstetricians" and objects to the hyper-ventilation (excessive intake of oxygen) which can result from the panting kind of breathing Lamaze had introduced.

Because the Lamaze teachings constitute a complete method, with a central Society (ASPO) devoted to the practice and to the training of teachers in the method, it has attracted much specific praise and also some criticism. Many believe that the rigorous demands of the training are excessive, rigid even, and do not emphasize strongly enough the wide variance in actual female experience in birth. A friend of mine who took a Lamaze preparation course several years ago says she felt betrayed, that no one had been able to get across the idea of just how much this was going to hurt, how hard and unpredictable the process could be. "The pain comes from out there somewhere," she was remembering. "You read all these books, and it's all very clear and nice, but then when your labor comes and it's different, you're lost . . . there needs to be some other way to prepare people."

Marjorie Karmel describes her surprise in hearing expectant mothers in a standard childbirth class (in the U.S.) carefully discussing and preselecting drugs for possible use during their labors: "Certainly [the teacher] was right when she said that no one should feel ashamed of taking drugs when she needed them. But it seems to me to be bad coaching to send you out on the field already resigned to defeat. I do think of labor as a contest. And I think it is worth taking the trouble to win." Yet the issue of medication is barely treated in Lamaze training. An easy-going delivery is envisioned while the possibility (except in emergency) that the woman would decide to ask for pain-killers is simply not dealt with. This is strong positive thinking, to be sure, but it sets up the real chance that if a woman loses her control, or decides she would like relief, she will emerge from the experience feeling she has failed. And, as Suzanne Arms points out in *Immaculate Deception*, the Lamaze method teaches the woman to separate herself from birth, rather than to become involved in all the basic sensuality of the experience.

In addition, many take issue with the insistence placed on the woman's staying alert, even if her coach has to use a cold washcloth to rouse her should she become sleepy between contractions. There is some feeling, too, that training for childbirth should begin well before the seventh month, which is when couples begin Lamaze classes.

Finally, the enthusiasm of Lamaze teachers and adepts focuses entirely on the achievement of the mother, on her heroic struggle to give birth successfully without pain. Delivery marks the completion of the Lamaze training. Many now feel that concerns about the baby have been entirely too much neglected. In the mid-70s another French obstetrician has introduced remarkable new ideas which are addressed to precisely that concern.

Leboyer: "Now, what about the suffering of the child?"

In a remarkably simple presentation, the French obstetrician Frederick Leboyer introduces his concept of *birth without violence*. For the past quarter-century, Dr. Leboyer has been delivering babies under the conditions he describes in the book of that name. That is, about 1000 of the 10,000 babies he has assisted into the world have enjoyed the special, compassionate care he learned to provide.

His premise is that "to be born is to suffer," that birth is violent (painful) and traumatic for the newborn, and that the task of obstetrics is to impose fewer demands on the baby, to remove the violence of the transition from intra-uterine life to life outside the womb. This includes removing all unnecessary interferences and requires that childbirth occur in an environment which combines the benefits of a hospital with the atmosphere of the home. Some key points in his method:

—the room should be dimmed (or darkened) at the time of delivery;
—the delivery room should be as silent as possible;
—the newborn should be placed on the mother's abdomen before the cord is cut;
—mother and newborn should greet each other first through the sense of touch;
—the newborn should be given a bath as his first independent experience.

Dr. Leboyer describes his own evolution in an interview segment on the videotape "Giving Birth," shown on National Educational Television, 1976.

His basic training, Leboyer says, was as a surgeon. He did much gynecological surgery, and, like most doctors in the 1940s and 1950s who had not digested Dr. Dick-Read's new-fangled ideas, was committed to the use of anesthesia to obliterate pain in the laboring mother. He was, he reports, "fascinated" by the miracle of drugs. Some of his patients, however, asked about painless natural childbirth. He knew nothing about it. For a long time he told them it was useless. The women insisted. "I had something new to learn . . . I had to go out of my way . . ." he remembers; he laughingly describes his own laziness. He decided to try to find out, and became acquainted with the work of Lamaze and especially Dick-Read: "I got some training and it opened my eyes."

"And," he continues, "once I could see for myself that definitely without any anesthesia, without any drug, a woman could really enjoy her delivery, which I had been witnessing for years and years as something really unbearable, I said, 'Oh yes, so this is suffering; so, in a way, suffering is something which we can do away with. It is not a fatality.' But then, being fully satisfied with the fact that we could free the mother from this suffering, suddenly I became aware of the suffering of the baby, and I said to myself, 'We've gone only half the way. We have completed only half the job. Now, what about the suffering of the child?' ''

He began to wonder about birth in the simplest, most direct way. What must it feel like to be born? His ability to imagine, to empathize with the sensations and even emotions of the emerging infant, combined with the medical knowledge and obstetric experience he had refined over years of practice, led to the insights which he shares in *Birth Without Violence*.

The book has three parts. Its language is as simple throughout as the quotations cited above. There are photographs in each part (forty in all, taken mostly by Dr. Leboyer).

Leboyer begins by introducing the notion that a newborn is a person, a preverbal person, to be sure, a person who is extremely sensitive and responsive but one whose perceptions of experience in the extra-uterine world are not yet arranged in the familiar way. (The newborn, he says in the videotape, "is a guest entering your house, in a way, so it should be treated like a guest.") He suggests we look closer at the standard photo of postpartum delight. The doctor looks pleased, pleased with "his" delivery. The mother is happy, she is justifiably relieved and proud, "her" delivery was successful. The father is a gratified man. But the baby. . . . We are offered a closeup of the infant, suspended by the heels, his face a mask of terror, eyes tight shut, mouth set in a howl, arms flailing blindly.

"Birth is a tidal wave of sensation, surpassing anything we can imagine. A sensory experience so vast we can barely conceive of it . . . rendered still more intense by contrast with what life was like before." Psychologists such as Carl Jung, Sigmund Freud, Otto Rank, Wilhelm Reich, and R.D. Laing (for a start) have theorized about the lasting effects on the psyche of the trauma of being born. Leboyer offers a direct, physical description of the events producing that trauma.

Regarding vision, for example, Leboyer guides us into the world of the infant. It is ture, says Leboyer, that the baby does not make pictures in its mind, but blind it is not. The baby perceives light while still in the womb. "If a woman more than six months pregnant is naked in the sunlight, the infant within her sees it as a golden haze." Suddenly this sensitive creature is thrust out of its dark cave into the glaring fluorescence of the modern hospital delivery room.

Similarly with hearing. A baby in the uterus perceives all the rumbling and grumbling of the digestive processes of the mother, the thump of her heart, the particular cadence of her voice, all muted. Then with birth suddenly comes the loud talk and metallic clanging of the modern birthing place.

And consider, implores Dr. Leboyer, what it is like to be touched, to be handled, for the *first* time. The skin of the newborn, used to being caressed by the soft fluid and the membranes in the womb, is suddenly and roughly slapped, then wrapped tightly in coarse, unfamiliar fabric.

Temperature alone is a terrible shock. The baby goes out of the body-temperature warmth and into the operating room, kept cool for the comfort of the attending personnel, onto the cold metal of the scale. Yet these shocks are nothing compared with the unbearable burn of the first breath of air. "For the infant coming into this world, the burning sensation of air entering the lungs surpasses every other horror." Leboyer compares the event with the reaction of clean lungs to that first deep draught of cigarette smoke. For the fetus in the uterus, oxygen-procuring has been mother's job. Via the placenta, she breathes for both. At birth this changes abruptly for the infant, who must now rely on inhalation and exhalation. Leboyer suggests that the painful transition can be eased, that right after the dangerous passage of birth the two systems can function simultaneously: bound to the mother still by the umbilical cord, the baby once born can have a few more minutes of settling into the new way—without violence.

In Part Two, Leboyer goes on to detail the remedy. His method for birth without violence centers around addressing the baby in its own language, the language of touch, soft and gentle, the language of love.

As soon as any possibility of danger is passed, why not dim the lights, he asks? Why not be silent, or whisper? In a *warm* room. Where better for the baby to be settled than on the mother's belly? It is soft, it has the familiar rise and fall. Without touching the infant's head (the most sensitive part, which has already undergone severe battering), the doctor or midwife should gently place the baby belly-to-belly on the mother.

Leboyer describes the agony for the newborn of being raised by the feet. The spinal column has been curved around for a long time; it should be allowed to straighten slowly, at its own pace. To suddenly hang the baby upside down robs him of all support, and forces his spine to straighten. To place the baby gently on his stomach, then turn him on the side which is relaxing to the limbs, and finally for a moment to place the baby on his back—this is the most merciful procedure. Leboyer suggests a soft, lovable massage by the mother's hands, to communicate with the child and to soften the pain.

The pictures that accompany this portion of *Birth Without Violence* are powerful support for the Leboyer thesis. These newborn babies look alert, comfortable, even relaxed.

Once the umbilical cord has pumped its last—and not until then—and has been cut, Leboyer advocates a simple procedure to give the

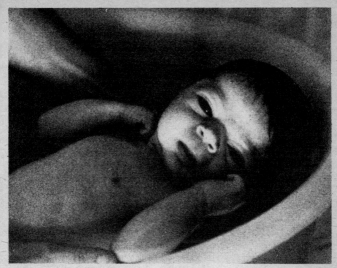

Leboyer Bath. This baby is being held in warm water just minutes after birth, to soothe and ease his transition from the uterine world to ours.

newborn the comfort of sensations that are familiar: place the child in body-temperature water. "Panic stops immediately." The infant relaxes. On the videotape a young couple gives birth to their fourth child at home. The room is quiet; the newborn boy gives several strong cries; then he is immersed in warm water, and the silence is profound. There is a genuine amazement in the face of the baby handled this way, as the photos in Dr. Leboyer's book show.

The bath is the detail of Leboyer's technique which has received the most criticism. For most hospitals the bath is impractical. Many say it puts too heavy a demand on the temperature-regulating system of the newborn. And it is perhaps sensorily confusing, rather than reassuring, to the newborn, once the transition out of the wet, warm life has already been accomplished.

Part Three of the book is recapitulation and coda. Leboyer assures us that if there is abnormality in the birthing, it must be dealt with in the fastest, most appropriate possible method. He assures us that each baby is different, that there are no ugly babies, "only those deformed by fear." And to the critic's first question—if birth is only a moment, why make such a fuss about it?—he answers: "At the end of our tale, I can only say one thing: 'Try.' "

Dr. Leboyer is now retired and spends two months of the year in India. While visiting that country he became acquainted with the ancient Indian art of infant massage. His second book, *Loving Hands*, is a presentation of that art in text and photographs. This work extends the concepts of *Birth Without Violence*, that we need to communicate directly and lovingly with our new children. Life in the womb was so rich, he reminds us. Most of all there was *movement* —supported, cradling, caressing movement. The massaging we can learn to give infants, he suggests, is as important for their growth as is the milk we feed them: "Being touched and caressed, being massaged, is food for the infant. . . . Deprived of this food, the name of which is love, babies would rather die. And they often do." (*Touching*, by the anthropologist/writer Ashley Montagu, addresses precisely this need in humans.)

The emphasis on compassion, always central to Leboyer's work, extends significantly the earliest modern ideas of a natural, painless childbirth. What Dick-Read taught us, and teaches us, is that the mother in childbirth can experience satisfaction, and joy, and freedom from fear, tension and pain. From Lamaze we are learning some specific physical and mental lessons for achieving this kind of childbirth. And in the empathy of Leboyer, among others, we have begun to wonder about communication with newborns, with babies, with children. Sensory and emotional communication is what the work of Klaus and Kennell (Chapter 1) investigates; it is at the foundation of the emergence of family-centered maternity care, of the struggle against routine hospital separation of baby and mother, and of the revival of breastfeeding. The development of these ideas is revolutionary in childbirth today, just like the fetal heart monitor and amniocentesis.

FURTHER THEORIES AND TECHNIQUES

There is a vast literature on natural childbirth. The basic ideas of Dick-Read and Lamaze have been reshaped, added to, updated, criticized and applied. In this section of the chapter we will take note of the work of several educators and writers, all of them women, whose reassuring and insightful books fortify our understanding of and preparation for the birth-giving experience. We will also touch upon the subject of mind control in preparation for labor.

Sheila Kitzinger

There is a certain wisdom in listening to what a mother who is also a long-time childbirth educator has to say about preparation for the event. Sheila Kitzinger studied childbirth in Jamaica, Mexico, and Germany as well as her native Great Britain. Formation of her method, the *psychosexual* method, began in 1958; the third edition of her book *The Experience of Childbirth,* was published in paperback in 1972. She is the mother of six children, several born at home.

"To anyone who thinks about it long enough," writes Kitzinger, "birth cannot simply be a matter of techniques for getting a baby out of one's body. It involves one's relationship to life as a whole." Accordingly she emphasizes the psychological aspects of pregnancy, labor, and postpartum adjustment, and attends greatly to the role of the husband in the process. Labor is viewed as "but one part" of a woman's "whole psychosexual life," which comprises "puberty, ovulation, menstruation, love-play and intercourse, pregnancy, labour, the involution of the uterus in the weeks following birth, breast feeding and menopause—there is a flow and rhythm about her life bound up with her sexuality."

Central to Kitzinger's view is harmony in mind and body. Her name for the kind of childbirth she teaches: Childbirth With Joy. It is not, in her view, "natural" childbirth; she prefers to speak of education for childbirth. The method she has developed continues to grow and change. This, it would seem, speaks well for its flexibility and adaptability.

Mind-body harmony, in Kitzinger's view, is attained through relaxation. Increasingly over the years she has integrated the idea of relaxation—which she considers an emotional experience involving one's image of one's body—into her teachings on prenatal preparation. Two major influences on her theories of relaxation are the idea of "sensory memory," derived from the Stanislavski method of teaching acting, and the work of Edmund Jacobson, whose 1939 book *Progressive Relaxation* was welcomed by Dick-Read as a "comprehensive addition to our knowledge and teaching upon the subject ."

Kitzinger's program of relaxation exercises is progressive, that is, it moves from one part of the body to another. Her program then leads from simpler kinds of sensory suggestions (imagine stepping into icy water) to more complex emotional ones ("you are lying in bed at night desperately wanting to cry and not wanting your husband to notice how unhappy you are"). First she instructs in relaxed breathing, how to feel heaviness in the limbs (checked by the husband if possible), and then relaxation of specific muscles in their turn, from the face on down. In this series of exercises differential relaxation is attempted, much like the Lamaze leg-with-alternate-arm tense/relax exercises. This ability, as we have noted, conserves energy.

Next she suggests ways to devise one's own exercises, physical experiences of stress-relaxation states which can be remembered and reconstructed. At the conclusion of each image, one is to relax.

From here she suggests recreating situations involving emotional conflict, such as the not-crying-in-bed example above. You learn to follow such a summoning-up with relaxation. Then you learn to *meet* it with relaxation. "Gradually," claims Kitzinger, "you'll develop a new neuro-muscular awareness. . . . It will be useful to you not only in labour, but in every situation in which you react with tension."

Kitzinger's next point is the touch-relax system. This bypasses verbal cues altogether in order to increase physical awareness of tension and release in a more direct way. Her experiments in this realm and in the use of massage were influenced in part, she says, by the movement of Esalen philosophy at the end of the 1960s. She has found that the touch-relax method has wider application than just during labor, with older women and with couples having sexual problems.

Touch-relax is a mutual exercise for husband and wife, and is simple enough. The woman contracts a part of the body, the shoulder perhaps; when she is ready her husband touches her on the contracted part, and immediately she releases the muscle, in the direction of the touch. Kitzinger suggests 14 or so specific parts of the body to try this with; her imagery is refreshing. In Exercise 14, for example, the woman is to press her buttocks together "as if she had a £5 note between them and someone was trying to take it away." The husband is to rest a hand on each buttock, and she then relaxes. Kitzinger explains the relevance of this exercise to labor: women often unconsciously resist when the pressure of the descending baby starts to be very strong; this pressure can make a woman feel as if the baby is going to split her apart, as if the baby fills all the pelvic region; the buttock muscles, among others, may contract to fight these feelings. Learning to relax those muscles, specifically, at a single touch, can be valuable.

Light massage of the small of the back, the lower spine, the buttocks, and inner thighs is recommended as part of the relaxation learning for husband and wife.

Kitzinger's treatment of breathing for labor is much less exacting than that of Lamaze; her emphasis is on the usefulness of establishing a rhythm to insure tranquility and to center attention. Her two recommended kinds of slow breathing and the one technique of quick, light breathing are similar to breathing methods already described in the Lamaze section of this chapter. Kitzinger views birthing as a central physical intensity which builds up, shifting by gears, and seems to dictate kind of breathing along the way.

One of Kitzinger's valuable offerings is the sexual/sensual awareness in birthing. Birth is the climax of a sexual process, and the mother has most success when she can open up, relax, and feel trusting. The urges and responses which her body expresses are primal: flushing, needing to push and grunting with the effort; supersensitivity between parts such as breasts and uterus, mouth and vagina. Kitzinger notes that many women who have retained control during second stage and avoided any numbing agents report orgasmic kinds of sensations as the baby emerges.

It requires for many of us quite an effort to open up this way in a hospital operating room among masked strangers and even friends. We have to plant ourselves squarely at the center of our body and go with it, tidiness and gentility set aside for the moment. Your body, if you have been training with it, is an authority with the doctor's medical know-how. Giving birth, like sexual intercourse, is an all-body involvement unique for each of us. It is about this involvement, in its demystified and pure form, that Ms. Kitzinger aims to educate us.

Erna Wright

Erna Wright is another Englishwoman with considerable childbirth education and experience, a clear writing style, and excellent advice. Her book *The New Childbirth* is like prenatal class in itself. My friend Julie, who gave birth to her first child in a little stone hospital in a tiny Welsh village, had no prenatal class or preparation except for this book, and she had a fine, calm, unmedicated delivery.

Wright has based her approach largely on the work of Dr. Dick-Read. She also studied with Pierre Vellay, Dr. Lamaze's colleague, in France. Wright modified the breathing techniques (the valuable "gear-shifting" imagery is hers), but her lessons are basically Lamaze-style, interspersed with topics like diet, the father's role, and the story of reproduction.

In childbirth preparation Wright stresses the need to practice in order to make the procedures as automatic as possible. She offers concrete suggestions to calm the distracted mind during labor—repeat a tune in your mind, in rhythm with the contraction. An example of her thinking and style: "As in any situation when you feel that life is too much for you" (here she is speaking of the helpless feelings of transition), "there is absolutely no reason for you to hang on grimly as though you were trying to prove something to yourself. Ask for an injection. You will only undermine your control of your nervous system if you lie there trying to perform unnecessary acts of heroism." And, from the same page: "Unfortunately, though, hospitals can be somewhat overgenerous with sedatives."

Lester Hazell, Constance Bean, and Valmai Elkins

Many good, overall childbirth education books, available in paper-back, present the basic aspects of a course of natural childbirth preparation: the story of labor and delivery, often with diagrams; a description of drugs and medical procedures; breathing techniques in straightforward or modified Lamaze form, often with diagrams indicating the shape and frequency of contractions in the various phases of labor; and basic comfort- and physical-fitness exercises for pregnancy, with their applicability to the laboring process.

These practical guides, including descriptions of hospital procedure, psychological insights, and reassuring advice, are indispensable to the expectant couple. I have found many women who particularly like *Commonsense Childbirth*, written by Lester Hazell, a mother and childbirth educator. At the end of her book she includes a section of frequently-asked questions and provides sensible, well-informed answers. Her style is direct and personal.

One example of the question-and-answer format: Question: *"I have often heard it said that women forget the pain of labor. If they really remembered, they wouldn't have any more babies. This is a frightening statement. Do you believe it?"* Hazell's response: "Certainly not. Such statements are made either by those who have never had a baby themselves or whose memory is distorted by nightmares produced by drugs. I have found that those who are the most realistic about the pain of childbirth are women who have large families. They neither minimize or exaggerate the pain. Discomfort is a small part of having a baby. Pretending it doesn't exist is bad, but statements tainted with sadism like the one above are inexcusable. You should watch the expression on the face of anyone who makes a negative remark about what is in store for you when you have your baby. The emotion you see reflected there will probably speak more eloquently than any refutation I can make."

The Boston-centered childbirth educator Constance Bean, author of the sound introductory work *Methods of Childbirth: A Complete Guide to Childbirth Classes and Maternity Care*, published a second book in 1977. *Labor & Delivery: An Observer's Diary* is a childbirth book of a different sort, and well worth the reading. This book presents information in narrative form, in a series of stories. In this format, childbirth experiences are related as they truly occur, as a cluster of facts, considerations, and conditions all hinged together. The economy of this presentation is one of the reasons it is recommended: the interrelationship of details is convincingly rendered. Using the experiential approach, Bean is conveniently able to present not only the standard information, but also such oft-ignored issues as patient permission for procedures.

Because *Labor & Delivery* is personal, we get profiles of many people from many corners of the childbirth world. One such portrait is that of a blind woman—blind because the oxygen level administered to premature newborns when she was born was too high—who gives birth at home. From the stance of observer, Bean draws a conclusion of sorts in her final paragraph: "Men and women need to learn about childbirth and to communicate with doctors, nurses and hospital administrators. They must demand knowledge of risks of routine intervention procedures. Women, with the support of their men, must select the kind of obstetrical care they wish and decide what they will accept."

A recent book from a Montreal childbirth educator, Valmai Howe Elkins, stresses the need for parents to be involved in planning for birth. In *The Rights of the Pregnant Parent*, Elkins gives her Lamaze-based method the name "Ultra-Prepared Childbirth." Elkins' point is that in addition to the essential physical and psychological preparations for childbirth, arranging the details with the hospital is a necessary other step in providing for a safe, satisfying birth experience. This book is full of pertinent data and narratives; its assertive, plain-speaking attitude makes good positive reading.

The emphasis Elkins puts on the importance of parents' making good doctor and hospital choices, the emphasis on using certain techniques to deal successfully with hospital routine, to, as she says, "get what you want from the obstetrical profession," is the tone of much childbirth education now. Such books can be guides of great value for parents who know what they want, or who are formulating a sense of what they want, but are not sure how to set about getting it. Elkins' list of Rights:

(1) the right to a supportive doctor;
(2) the right to a healthy baby;
(3) the right to childbirth education;
(4) the right to a shared birth experience;
(5) the right to a childbirth with dignity;
(6) the right to family-centered maternity care.

Clearly, some of these rights are more readily realized than others. Economic and educational differences among us partly determine how good are our chances of giving birth to a healthy baby. Liberal, family-centered hospital facilities may be more convenient to upper-class neighborhoods, and/or may price themselves in those brackets only. Medical assistance usually provides minimal care at the large, local hospital; obstacles to claiming the above listed rights in such a setting may be nearly insurmountable. We will discuss this issue more in Chapter 5.

Elizabeth Noble

The best presentation I have seen of physical exercises for pregnancy, labor, and the postpartum period is *Essential Exercises For the Child-bearing Year* by Elizabeth Noble, a physical therapist who has specialized in obstetrics and gynecology for many years. A handsome, focused book, it does not attempt to give a general philosophy of the issues in childbirth, but attends rather to physiological details. Noble's attitude is clear without being strident: for reasons of health the mother who prepares herself physically is increasing her chances of an uncomplicated birth and speedy recovery. The directions for muscular restoration after birth are especially useful, as is the section about Caesareans and recovery from them.

The exercises in this book are designed to: (1) promote a general limbering of the body, which makes the work of giving birth less taxing; (2) help in developing good muscle tone, for increased efficiency in labor and quicker recovery of muscle tone afterward; (3) teach specific muscle control to facilitate labor and delivery. Noble's view emphasizes prevention and control. The pelvic floor, the abdominal muscles, and the back muscles, sites of particular strain in pregnancy and labor, receive special attention. Also—a valuable feature—Noble indicates what *not* to do.

Noble's chapter on relaxation is an exemplary treatment of the subject. She teaches a few simple exercises to practice with a partner during pregnancy, emphasizes basic muscle control and conscious muscle release, more and more specifically. Noble expresses the general benefit of such preparation: ''Gaining skills in relaxation pays off with greater poise and emotional serenity as well as such physiological benefits as reduced blood pressure (since better circulation is allowed when the muscles are free from undue tension). With bodily tensions reduced, there are fewer cramped muscles, headaches, backaches, and insomnia. Learning this art—learning to unwind—is of value for the rest of our lives, whatever our age, sex, or occupation.''

Breathing directions are similarly clear and detailed.

Noble explains succinctly in anatomical and physiological terms the way to most benefit your labor as it is occurring. Little hints emerge as major advice; there is the frequent reminder, for instance, of how tension in muscles of the vagina and tension in the mouth and jaw are closely related.

Line drawings in her book illustrate the geography of the entire pelvic cavity, from the perineum at the bottom to the diaphragm at the top.

Hypnosis, meditation, and mind control

The classical form of hypnosis, where the subject is maneuvered into a trancelike state by a trained practitioner, does not seem to be harmonious with other aspects of prepared childbirth. Dr. Dick-Read rejected the hypotheses of some of his critics who assumed his natural childbirth successes depended upon his establishing this kind of occult power relationship with women in labor. But hypnotic techniques can have value in learning relaxation during the preparatory months.

I asked my obstetrician about hypnosis, a technique which he used for years and which was part of the training I had with him during the last four to six weeks of my pregnancy in 1969. The main component in his version was complete bodily relaxation, the progressive kind (in the Jacobson tradition), where one part of the body after another is talked into relaxation by the attendant. Perhaps the term best describing this state is suggestibility, that mentally alert, physically inactive, opened-up condition we have almost all experienced at some time—after orgasm, slowly drifting off to sleep, during meditation. Though it is not trancelike (I clearly remembered our sessions afterward), the mind does create pleasant pictures as suggested. I even now remember how refreshed and calm I always felt as I left the office. This type of relaxation-hypnosis does not contain any hypnotic suggestion about behavior during labor.

Another component in learning this kind of relaxation is verbal signals. A person in the aware, relaxed, meditative state (characterized in the brain by waves of the sort called alpha) is mentally tuned-up in a state of mind receptive to learning new responses. The woman's husband (or coach) can develop with her (as Kitzinger describes) verbal signals and touch signals which will stimulate certain physical responses, like instantly stopping pushing when that is called for, or relaxing the jaw and the perineum. These signals can be practiced during preparation for labor, coordinated with breathing.

In the opinion of the obstetrician cited above, the benefit of hypnosis in preparation for childbirth is just like the benefit of a Lamaze or Dick-Read-like preparation. Indeed Lamaze training and hypnosis both aim to provide new learning pathways, new stimulus-response patterns for the time when the stimulus is a uterine contraction. On the other hand, William S. Kroger, M.D., author of *Childbirth With Hypnosis,* believes that Dick-Read's technique was correct but did not go far enough. Dick-Read's approach treats the fear/tension/pain syndrome in the conscious mind, whereas hypnosis *"invokes the conviction* that fears and hidden anxieties will not lead to painful sensations" (Kroger's italics). To block the mental perception of pain, states Kroger, is the aim of the hypnosis.

Regarding post-hypnotic amnesia, Kroger suggests that the subject herself request either partial or total forgetfulness to follow the trancelike period.

For Kroger, hypnotic suggestibility is rooted in self-concentration, self-discipline. For their part, Lamaze teachers insist on practice to insure this concentration. A self-discipline course known as Alpha Mind Control, like the teachings of the Transcendental Meditation (TM) movement, works to achieve the same goal: to lead people into a state of relaxation and suggestibility, and then instill positive direction for the thus-released energy. Ultimately, whether the voice that guides you belongs to a physician, hypnotist, class instructor, meditation teacher, your husband, or yourself is of less importance than the gradual achievement of overall bodily relaxation accompanied by mental alertness and a state of suggestibility.

What I have read about self-hypnosis, apart from the work done in the Soviet Union early this century, makes it also sound in effect much like other meditative and relaxation techniques and like some of Kitzinger's exercises in particular. That is the self-hypnosis which Leslie LeCron describes in the chapter on childbirth in his book *The Complete Guide to Hypnosis.*

The idea of meditation has been with us for a long time, all around the world. Although techniques now have different names and are taught in unique ways, the aim is one: to free the mind and body from tenseness and anxiety, to promote tranquility, to release natural energy for our use and growth: *to achieve relaxation.*

A good childbirth education class teaches relaxation. Yoga teaches relaxation. Alpha Mind Control teaches relaxation. Meditation instruction is instruction in relaxation. The physical and psychological importance of relaxation in humans is enormous—that much is clear. As a tool of preparation for labor it becomes the beginning point and ending point of breathing and muscular exercises which further prepare the mind and body to give birth consciously. In preparation for childbirth, relaxation attained through meditation or otherwise is an end worth achieving by the father as well as the mother.

Russell is a meditation teacher, employed at a Community Mental Health Center where he teaches staff and clients alike. He is also a new father, whose daughter was born recently at Booth Maternity Center in Philadelphia. Russell and his wife Jackie undertook a Lamaze preparation and also sat in on some of the preparation classes at Booth. I asked Russell if meditation had come up as a prenatal topic of discussion or practice at the classes he went to. He told me that in one class the women were practicing total relaxation (which is, in fact a yoga posture), being checked by their husbands for relaxation level. Russell suggested to the teacher that *the husbands* do the relaxation with the wives. They did, and they reported that this had been of positive benefit to the couple: the effort of the relaxing woman is helped if her support and coach is able to stay physically relaxed and mentally alert and open with her.

3

Drugs, Devices, Surgeries, Procedures

Pain in labor, its origins and its character, has been described in the opening chapter. Chapter 2 introduced some ideas about painless childbirth and some methods for preparing to experience birth with as little discomfort and as little interference as possible. Here we will consider the medications used to decrease or remove discomfort in labor, and then describe some of the devices and procedures—chemical, surgical, mechanical, and otherwise—that are regularly employed in hospital births and are less frequently associated with maternity-center and home deliveries.

Attempts to relieve discomfort in labor and delivery and to prevent tragedy in childbirth go back as far as we have stories. In some cultures long ago a woman experiencing difficulty in labor might have been shaken up in a blanket, or hung from a tree, or jumped upon to help her get the baby out. Spells might have been said over her. Music, dancing, or wailing perhaps accompanied her toil. In most times and places she would be attended by a woman specializing in remedies and treatments during birth. When midwives began to be persecuted with witches and *as* witches in Western Europe, however, their effort was punishable by death at the stake.

The use of drugs to relieve pain in childbirth began with herbs, opium, and alcohol. By the sixteenth century obstetrics emerged as a medical specialty. New techniques for the management of labor began to appear. Forceps, techniques of version (manipulating the unborn within the uterus), episiotomy, safe Caesarean section, induction of labor, and various forms of medication have all been developed and refined within the last 400 years. When Queen Victoria ignored the prevailing religious creed and accepted chloroform in 1853 for the birth of her son Leopold, a new era of anesthesia in childbirth began.

Now we are in another new era: that of high technology, including prenatal surgery, amniocentesis, fetal heart monitoring, and a staggering variety of medications.

Today, only about 10% of labors in our culture proceed without some level of obstetric interference. With the achievements of technology and pharmacology, however, comes a recognition of the hazards involved in much obstetrical practice (just as environmental pollution has in recent years been teaching us much about the limitations of industrial progress). As a result, drugs and medical procedures are now being scrutinized by concerned parents, nurses, midwives, physicians, and researchers to reevaluate the wisdom and determine the safety of their use. The effect of drugs and routine procedures *on the newborn* especially has become a subject of intense investigation.

Unfortunately, drugs are not always well enough tested before they enter the mainstream of medical practice. Mothers who took the sedative/hypnotic thalidomide during their pregnancy a number of years ago do not need to be reminded. Unfortunately, too, the dangers of a drug or procedure are not always spelled out even when they are known or suspected. As a consumer of gynecological and obstetrical medicine, it is your right and your need to learn as much as you can about what substances might be put into you, and what procedures might be performed on you.

Persevere in your effort to know; it is not easy. Most hospitals, like most doctors, have their routines. Usually understaffed, always trying to do the best they can under the given conditions, they may not want to take the time to make an exception of your case. But it is your baby, it is your body; what happens in those hours while you are giving birth can profoundly affect your life and health and the life and health of your child. So persevere. As pleasantly and understandingly as you can, request the information you wish, and make clear your own needs and fears.

If your labor becomes dysfunctional, or if a complication arises which in your doctor's opinion warrants serious intervention, of course he or she will be the one to decide what medical or surgical intervention is necessary. We do not pretend to know emergency obstetrics. We can only bring with us knowledge of and confidence in our bodies, and a willingness to cooperate intelligently with medical assistance. We can avoid the powerlessness and danger of forced labor by educating ourselves, by preparing, and by working honestly with our birth attendant(s).

The most complete and clear criticisms of the way American obstetrics manages birth come from Suzanne Arms, in *Immaculate Deception*, and from Doris Haire, in *The Cultural Warping of Childbirth*. Their sense of outrage, of human concern, of serious criticism supported by scientific fact, marks these works as critical to our evaluation of our own experiences and to our effort to bring about the needed changes.

There are, of course, many reasons to be thankful to the obstetrics profession. One baby in 20 would not survive his birth if the technique of Caesarean section had not been developed. Thanks to the judicious use of forceps, mothers have been spared exhaustion and babies have been spared damage that might have resulted from prolonged labor, breech presentation, multiple fetuses, or otherwise stressful labors. New monitoring techniques are able to detect fetal difficulties and thereby preserve the health, and sometimes the life, of the unborn. The one-in-thirty whose prenatal life is threatened by postmaturity, placental insufficiency, or some form of dysfunctional labor, benefits from careful administration of labor-stimulating chemicals. And multitudes of mothers are reassured, soothed, and aided in their laboring by medications and anesthetic agents applied at the right time and in the right dose.

Why then is the emphasis in this chapter on the hazards of medications and procedures in obstetrics today?

Benefits of analgesics and anesthetics do not take long in the telling: these substances remove or diminish pain felt by the laboring woman. Once, when we thought the fetus inviolate in its uterine home, the emphasis in obstetrics was on developing more and more drugs and procedures to benefit the mother. Now we know that the placenta is not a chemical barrier. The risks of analgesics and anesthetics are risks to the health of the baby and sometimes also to the safety of the mother. These dangers are complicated, and we are only still discovering them. These risks vary with dosage, with the woman's size and tolerance, and with her psychological condition. Further, there are hazards in the method of administration, in the timing, and in the combined effects if more than one drug is being used. The story of hazards is more complicated, more recent, more urgent to tell than the reassuring story we already know—how drugs reduce pain and how oxytocin and forceps get the baby out quicker.

Once childbirth entered the hospital it became the province of Medicine. The medicine of no other culture leaps so enthusiastically as ours into a chemical and technological management of life. Often this occurs without regard for the consequences. Now it is our challenge to admit to these consequences, become educated, and express our preferences about the way *our* babies will be born.

MEDICATIONS

There are two major classes of medication for pain relief in labor and delivery, analgesics and anesthetics. Analgesics induce a state of insensibility to pain without loss of consciousness. Anesthetics induce a loss of sensation to an area or part of the body, or to the entire body.

Analgesics

These are drugs which raise the threshold of pain, that is, inhibit the receiving of pain stimuli; they also cause drowsiness. In childbirth analgesics are used principally during the first stage of labor, to "take the edge off" the discomfort of contractions, especially those of transition.

Demerol, a trademark of meperidine (synthetic morphine) is the most widely used analgesic in childbirth. It is injected intravenously (into the vein, I.V.) or, less commonly, intramuscularly; its effects are immediate. The resulting physical sensation is one of floating, or being far away. Demerol relaxes, and induces grogginess.

Many obstetricians believe that Demerol or its equivalent is exactly the right drug for labor; it is simple to administer, it does not knock the woman out completely, it does help relaxation, and it does not produce painful aftereffects. An estimated 80% to 90% of deliveries in Great Britain include the use of meperidine.

Demerol affects the baby, too. Drugs (including caffeine, nicotine, and alcohol) enter the infant's system instantly via the placenta. Once the placenta was referred to as the placental barrier: now we know that it is no barrier at all. Whatever the mother takes into her system she shares with her unborn child. The Society for Research in Child Development published a report in 1970 which expresses this clearly: "Virtually all obstetric medication—nausea remedies, diuretics, sedatives, muscle relaxants, analgesics, regional anesthesia and general anesthetics—tend to rapidly cross the placenta and alter the fetal environment as they enter the circulatory system of the unborn infant within seconds or minutes of administration to the mother."

A dose of medication large enough to make a grown woman drowsy may be expected to noticeably affect the baby; and the closer to delivery the drug is administered, the more marked its effects on the infant. The mother's body relaxes as the meperidine solution trickles in through her hand; her breathing slows down, her blood pressure drops somewhat. These changes register in the fetus, too. Although a standard dose of meperidine is not considered by most obstetricians to be dangerous to the fetus, such a dose does reduce blood supply, and hence oxygen supply, to the uterus. Many doctors and institutions are giving smaller doses and having successful results—with Demerol, 25 mg gives relief but leaves mother much less groggy and affects the baby correspondingly less than the 75-100 mg which used to be the standard dose several years ago.

The vital sign most critical to watch in a baby being born and just born is the delivery of oxygen to its system. Food is not an issue at this time in the baby's life; actual nutrition does not begin with an infant for at least some hours after parturition. But oxygen is essential. In the uterus, and during birth, the fetus receives its oxygen from the mother through the placenta via the umbilical cord. This system continues to function until the cord is cut and the lungs inflate with air on their own. Any interference with the supply of oxygenated blood passing from mother to fetus is potentially dangerous. Any technique which could cramp the cord and thus decrease oxygen to the fetus is dangerous. Any state of the uterus itself which prevents the placenta from delivering blood to the cord is likewise life-threatening.

Blood carrying oxygen must get to the baby's brain or the brain will start losing some of its functions. How much oxygen deprivation can the baby sustain? In *Safe Alternatives in Childbirth* (published by the NAPSAC—National Association of Parents and Professionals for Safe Alternatives in Childbirth), Doris Haire addresses the question: "It is important that you realize that no one knows the degree of oxygen deprivation an unborn or newborn infant can tolerate before he or she sustains permanent brain damage. It is likely that most American women would not be so quick to demand pharmacological relief from their discomfort if they were advised of the potential dangers of the drugs to the integrity of their baby's brain and its future intellectual functioning."

Analgesics, then, should be considered from more than one point of view. Yes, they aid the mother in relaxing and in not noticing pain, while still leaving her more or less conscious; but the consequent drop in her blood pressure means that the fetus is having to get along with less oxygen than is optimal. This does not automatically mean catastrophe, we should hasten to add. It is simply a known medical fact which should be added in with the complex set of considerations in making a decision about analgesic drugs during labor.

Yet it should also be added that the effects of drugs on the fetus do not have to be catastrophic in order to justify re-evaluating routine administration. A complete postpartum evaluation of the newborn's health will include more than just the critical signs of the Apgar scoring.

Studies show that a baby whose mother received Demerol or some stronger analgesic is less active after birth than a baby who has not received the same drug via its mother. The sucking reflex is diminished in such babies, as is visual attention. Concerning respiration, *Our Bodies, Ourselves* reports a study in which less than 2% of babies delivered of nonmedicated mothers had delayed respiration, while 35%-67% of babies born of sedated mothers had a delay. The delay or the depression in respiration in such cases is called "serious." And, examining the ability of newborns to process information, research from 1974 concludes that there is a clear difference between infants of mothers who were given meperidine and those whose mothers were not. A difference of the same kind exists in infant response to cuddling.

Moreover, the dynamics of the sedated state may be counterproductive to the best efforts of the laboring woman. One Lamaze-trained mother describes her analgesic experience this way: "At first I argued with the doctor, assuring him that I could go on for hours without taking any drugs, but he convinced me that a tiny dose of Demerol would be helpful to our efforts. It wasn't! It did nothing to relieve the powerful contractions—it merely fouled up my ability to concentrate, to catch each contraction before it caught me. I felt very much like a drunk trying to walk a straight line."

Another possible effect of the use of sedatives in childbirth is that labor may subsequently need to be speeded up with an oxytocic stimulant; and if the labor is slowed down in second stage, forceps may be called for. The point here is simply that an otherwise innocent touch of something to "take the edge off" the discomfort of contractions may bring with it a series of other drugs and/or procedures, each with its own risks. It is important to be aware that in taking medication one may be stepping on a medical carousel which even with the best of professional attendance can go whirling quite out of control—not necessarily *will*, but, in some small percentage of cases, *could*.

Also used in early labor and stronger than narcotic-sedatives (such as Demerol) is the class of analgesics known as barbiturates; Seconal and Nembutal are popular trademarks. Barbiturates produce sleep; their use close to delivery may not be wise. For all the cautions mentioned above regarding meperidine, the same is even more true of barbiturates. These substances are stored in the midbrain of the newborn, and their effects last at least one week. Quite a task it is for the barely-formed physical systems of a seven-pound human to have to cope with a dose of depressive adult drugs.

Tranquilizers, such as Miltown® (meprobamate) or Valium® (diazepam), are also used to help the mother relax. Occasionally they are administered with another, stronger analgesic. In reduced version they carry the same kinds of hazards as the stronger analgesics. Furthermore, a British study from the late 1960s shows that Valium interferes noticeably with the newborn's ability to fight the stress of cold.

Anesthetics: general and local

The other major class of medication for pain relief is anesthetics, which are of two kinds. Those which block sensation in a specific

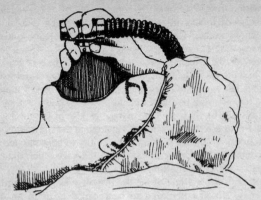

General Anesthetic: Inhalant. General anesthetic is sometimes given this way just as the baby's head is crowning; the woman herself may administer it.

location of the body, causing numbness, are the local, or regional, anesthetics (also called conduction anesthetics). General anesthetics are those which block consciousness altogether.

General anesthetics come usually in inhalant form. James Simpson, a Scottish physician, is credited with having discovered the use of chloroform in childbirth. This was in 1847, after some earlier attempts with ether. Despite immediate protest that the use of anesthesia constituted a tampering with Divine Order, the use of the gas continued and in 1853 received official recognition when Queen Victoria of England accepted chloroform for the birthing of her seventh child, Leopold.

Taking gas then became the fashion. As recently as the 1940s and 1950s women routinely accepted this general anesthetic, turning the whole birthing business over to the doctor and his attendants. In 1941 my mother went into the hospital to have her first baby. As soon as labor was well established and becoming ''heavy'' (transition, probably) she was given an inhalant and was knocked out. An hour or two later she awoke, she says, black and blue on wrists and ankles, miserably sick, and aching all over: ''sandbagged'' is her description. She says it took hours to feel any tenderness for or recognition of the screaming infant someone handed to her and said was her son. Obstetricians and parents have made this knockout method of childbirth a thing of the past. Inhalants are sometimes used, self-administered with a small face mask, but nowadays it is just for individual moments such as the peak of transition or the instant of crowning. This use brings relief, and does not appear to impair the fetus. It is a popular choice in Sweden.

Gases used as general anesthetic agents include Fluoromar® (Fluroxene), Fluothane® (halothane), Penthrane® (methoxyflurane), Trilene® (trichloroethylene), cyclopropane with oxygen, ethyl ether (very uncommon), and oxygen with sodium Pentothal® (thiopental sodium, a barbiturate). Nitrous oxide (laughing gas), used by dentists since 1772, also is used.

These drugs affect the mother's entire system. Beginning within minutes of being administered they have a correspondingly greater effect on the more sensitive system of the newborn. The baby of a mother so thoroughly drugged comes out limp, needing considerable help to begin breathing. Such a baby demands special observation for hours after birth.

General anesthesia must be administered by highly trained personnel; the mother requires constant watching. It is important that the mother's stomach be completely empty. Under a general anesthesia in the supine position, a person whose stomach is not completely empty risks vomiting and possibly choking to death from the vomitus before she can be saved. A 1969 obstetrical report claims that this danger is one of the reasons that obstetrical anesthesia is close to being the fourth leading cause of maternal mortality in childbirth.

A unique general anesthetic, developed specifically for discomfort in childbirth, is the hallucinogenic/amnesic medication known as scopolamine or "twilight sleep." Hailed in the early part of the century as the savior of womankind, used widely some decades ago, it is still occasionally administered in combination with morphine and/or other sedatives. Dr. Henry Smith Williams, an enthusiastic proponent of the new miracle, thus explained in 1914: "Stated in the fewest words, this method consists essentially in the hypodermic administration of certain drugs, given just at the incipiency of the acute pains of childbirth, and calculated to render the patient oblivious of the pains—or, to be quite accurate, to modify her consciousness in such a way that she has no recollection of suffering when the ordeal is over." Williams is accurate; the actual sensation of pain is not reduced by the drug, although the memory is. The woman experiences a restless, half-sleeping state which may include hallucinations. Attending personnel tend to assume that a woman so treated is basically unconscious and do not give analgesic relief. The woman under twilight sleep often has to be strapped down to prevent her thrashing from injuring herself and the baby. After delivery, the mother sleeps off the drug's effects and the whole experience is buried in unconsciousness. Nonanalgesic, it has been described as "the only drug that childbirth educators recommend that women not have."

There are obstetricians who continue to use this drug, despite its declining reputation. Dr. Arthur Gorbach, for instance, in *Pregnancy, Birth, & the Newborn Baby* (by the Boston Children's Medical Center, 1972), makes these statements: "Today, scopolamine is often given with barbiturates and tranquilizers for analgesia. In the doses used, these drugs do not depress the baby's respiration. Some people are afraid the drugs will harm the baby. You need not worry. There has been enough experience with them that your doctor knows what the safe and reasonable doses are." Gorbach recognizes some hazards, but concludes: "In spite of the drawbacks, however, most women find the combination of scopolamine, barbiturates, and tranquilizers very satisfactory."

In light of considerable research, Gorbach is clearly in the minority position. Research by Scanlon in 1974 concludes that the combination of scopolamine and sedatives creates "severe neonatal depression." Other studies could be cited, but for me the final argument against the use of twilight sleep rests in the nature of the woman's experience. Is it, indeed, very satisfactory?

There will be differences among women when considering a drug experience like this. My reaction to the idea of twilight sleep is decidedly negative; to me it seems like a combination of just the wrong effects: the pain is undiminished and the memory of the event is gone. A mother has described this as "the sort of medication male doctors would invent"—an unkind characterization, but based on the truth that only childbearing women can evaluate the subjective experience of birth and of the procedures and medications which accompany it. If I am going to accept medication to relieve my discomfort in labor, I would rather it (a) diminish the pain, and (b) leave me with a memory of the event.

Dr. John Franklin of Booth Maternity Center speaks of "price tags" in evaluating medical procedures. The psychic price tag on scopolamine is too high for me, but it may not be too high for someone else, who perhaps puts highest value on being able to escape the pain of birthing.

Characteristic of all general anesthesia, whether the mother is conscious or not, is a diminished *ability* to participate in the birthing process.

Local anesthetics (or *regional* or *conduction* anesthetics) are area-specific numbing agents which are injected into the body once, or continuously with the use of a catheter (tube). They make numb the area of the body around or below the injection by blocking nerve impulses from there to the brain. Regional anesthetics, which include spinals, caudals, saddle blocks, and epidural blocks, are injected into the spinal column; paracervical blocks are injected into the cervix; pudendal blocks, used for delivery only, are injected into the sides of the birth canal to deaden the sensation of the vagina and perineum. The drugs injected include a whole class of sensation-numbers such as Xylocaine® (lidocaine), Novocain® (procaine hydrochloride), Carbocaine® (mepivacaine), Metycaine® (piperocaine), and most recently Nesacaine® (chloroprocaine).

The regional anesthetic which affects the largest area is the *spinal*, in which the drug is injected after transition directly into the cerebrospinal fluid at the location called the spinal subarachnoid space. (The spinal column has three membranes covering it, of which the arachnoid is innermost; cerebrospinal fluid flows between the arachnoid membrane and the pia mater, the central membrane; the dura mater is the outermost). The injection is administered to the lower spine of the woman in a sitting position. Within minutes she will be numb from that point down to the knees. One injection will usually maintain anesthesia through delivery.

Spinals were welcomed as a procedure for obtaining pain relief and yet retaining consciousness; they had wide use in the 1940s and 1950s, and into the 1960s. The decline in usage of spinals reflects our accumulating evidence of the problems attendant upon their use.

This method of anesthesia slows down labor significantly. The uterus relaxes, contractions lose their full force and downward pressure, blood pressure may drop and thereby reduce the oxygen supply to the unborn child. The mother loses all sensation in the birthing part of her body. The spinal also affects the motor impulses of the treated area, so that the woman is not only numb to the knees, she is paralyzed. It is just about impossible for her to push the baby out; forceps are often necessary as a substitute for her muscle work. Further, it seems that spinal anesthesia leads to incomplete rotation of the fetal head in delivery, which also increases the likelihood of forceps use.

Other risks of the spinal and possible attendant procedures: need for oxytocin to accelerate the depressed labor; artificial rupturing of the membranes, which is done to be certain the baby is presenting its head and is not stuck in a transverse position, as sometimes happens with the slowing down of uterine activity; and use of the fetal heart monitor to check the baby's reaction to the anesthetic. Constant monitoring of the woman on a spinal is necessary to check for blood pressure drop (hypotension); should this occur she can be given intravaneous hydrating solution and be turned on her side to take pressure off the major artery supplying blood to the uterus.

For the mother, the spinal in some cases results in a severe head-

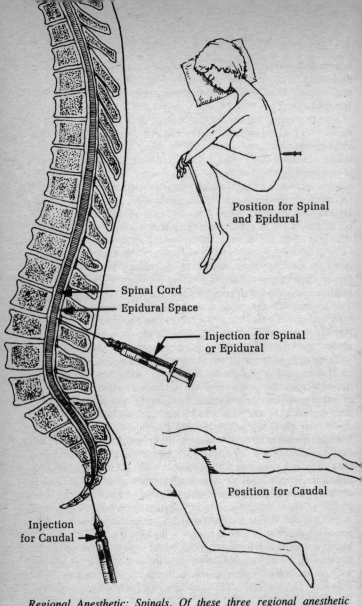

Spinal Cord
Epidural Space

Injection for Spinal or Epidural

Position for Spinal and Epidural

Position for Caudal

Injection for Caudal

Regional Anesthetic: Spinals. Of these three regional anesthetic choices, the spinal is the only one given in a single injection; the other two are administered continually via a catheter, after the initial injection.

ache lasting several days after delivery. The use of finer-gauge needles has in recent years lessened this threat; for those mothers who do not escape the headache, the immediate postpartum period is wretched.

Spinals have given way recently to the other, less severe, forms of regional block. *Saddle block,* also called "little" spinal, is injected into the lower back, but is more precise and less wide in its effect than the spinal. The area treated is just the area which would touch a saddle if one were riding a horse.

Medication for *caudal blocks,* first used in 1901, is injected into the sacral canal, below the lumbar vertebrae and above the coccyx. Instead of being administered in one injection, the caudal block is continuous: a plastic tube called a catheter keeps the drug flowing in at a slow, constant rate. This can be begun at about 5 cm of dilation.

Maternal hypotension (low blood pressure) is a possible complication in caudal blocks. Improper placement of the needle also constitutes a risk. On rare occasions the anesthetic has been known to be injected by mistake into the baby's head; this can cause fetal death. The woman with a caudal block requires constant supervision. As with the spinal, slowed labor is a potential outcome, increasing the possibility of added procedures and, in turn, the risks described above.

The *epidural,* like the caudal, is applied continuously, higher in the spine than the caudal but not mixing with the cerebrospinal fluid. Like the other regional blocks it slows labor, bringing with it the likelihood of a forceps delivery (in *The Rights of the Pregnant Parent* Elkins estimates 75%). There is, further, the risk of puncture, and of spinal-style headache, if application is incorrect. The epidural is the current "favorite" among obstetricians who, though supportive of noninterference, like nevertheless to have available a routine pain relief. It used to be Demerol; now it is epidural. In Sweden, where a whiff of gas at an appropriate moment has tended to be the only medication commonly resorted to, hospitals are now advertising the presence of an epidural-trained anesthesiologist on round-the-clock duty.

Some studies show decreased muscle tone and strength for some period of time in a baby delivered under epidural anesthesia. Dr. Murray Enkin of Toronto also reports depressing of the sucking response and of muscle reflexes several days after birth conducted with an epidural anesthetic.

Despite the glowing reports of this drug, these cautions are useful. Low blood pressure, as with caudal blocks, often occurs in the mother following epidural. Then oxytocin, forceps, and episiotomy often follow. Elkins estimates that 80% of deliveries in Montreal hospitals are under epidural.

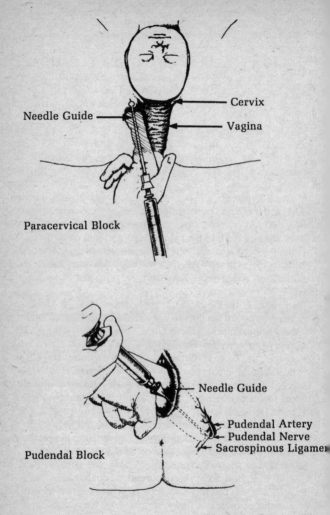

Cervix

Needle Guide

Vagina

Paracervical Block

Needle Guide

Pudendal Artery
Pudendal Nerve
Sacrospinous Ligamen

Pudendal Block

Local anesthetic: Paracervical blocks are used in first-stage labor to numb the cervix as it dilates; a dose lasts one to two hours, and may be repeated. Pudendal blocks are given for delivery and episiotomy; they numb the vagina and perineum.

There are two other local blocks used regularly. Some women during first-stage labor are given a *paracervical block*, whereby a needle injects anesthesia directly into the cervix on both sides, aimed away from the baby's head or other presenting part. This numbness lasts from 40 minutes to an hour and can be renewed. Research done in Israel in 1971 shows that paracervical block is the cause of "severe changes in the fetal heart rate in 35% of cases . . . changes which are often followed by prolonged acidosis of the fetus with a significant number of depressed neonates" (Suzanne Arms). The study concludes with the words: "fetal depression, even if apparently reversible, might later affect the motor and intellectual development of the child." Apgar scores of 6 or less, reports Doris Haire, are almost three times more numerous among infants whose mothers had paracervical blocks than among the control group.

Pudendal block is anesthetic injected either into the buttocks, aimed toward the pelvic region, or into the vagina. Its purpose is to remove the sensation during those moments when the baby is emerging. It is used also for the doing and repairing of the episiotomy.

Usually the pressure of the baby's head on the perineum while the vaginal opening is stretching is a natural anesthetic; indeed, most mothers report that the second, expulsive stage of labor is the least painful, most satisfying part of the entire process. Yet the pudendal block is one of the most routinely administered of all the childbirth medications. This minor anesthetic has been found to cause a "persistent decrease in oxygen saturation in the newborn during the first thirty minutes of postpartum observation."

The point, once again, is *not* that anesthetic and analgesic medications lack merit; they can be of great benefit to the woman in labor and to the entire laboring process—that much we have known for a long time. But while the benefits are, for the most part, obvious, the hazards associated with medication during labor have in many cases not been recognized. Our increasing awareness of the risks involved comes primarily from two sources (1) obstetric technology, which has taught us much about intrauterine life and fetal sensitivities; and (2) the recognition that the placenta is not a barrier to the passage of substances from the mother to the fetus.

Participating responsibly in the decision-making for the way your labor will be managed requires that you be aware of any potential danger to you or your baby. Many ifs and unknowns come into play. To be sure, a fine balance of considerations must enter into any decision to medicate the woman in labor. But how about the *baby* in labor? Dr. Leboyer, perhaps the most poetic statesman in the field, is hardly alone in this concern. The case against medication, militantly expressed in *Immaculate Deception,* involves a radical shift in emphasis from pain relief in the mother to well-being in the newborn: "How many times must it be said?" writes Suzanne Arms: *"Drugs get to the baby. Drugs adversely affect the baby. Drugs may permanently damage the baby* [Arms' italics]. Any doctor who tells his patient that any drug used for any reason—including tranquilizers, sedatives, caudals, epidurals, saddle blocks, paracervical blocks, spinals, generals, or whatever—will not affect the baby is telling her an untruth: no drug has been proven not to affect the baby, and therefore, as (Geoffrey) Chamberlain says, 'No drug can be said to be absolutely blame free.' Why risk it? Why not turn the 'just-in-case' game back to the doctor and say, 'No, just in case *this* drug has an effect on my baby that you don't know about yet, I won't take it.''

It is the other side of the coin, and it is worth examining.

DEVICES AND PROCEDURES

Prepping, enema, and I.V.

These are three virtually routine practices in North American hospital births. None is horrendous, none brings excessive hazard. Each may have a definite usefulness; yet each is, in its way, a discomfort, and each is often unnecessary.

Prepping (preparation) is the name given to the practice of shaving or clipping the mother's pubic hair when she appears at the hospital labor floor. The reason for the procedure is cleanliness; however, Doris Haire reports that shaved women actually have a slightly higher incidence of infection than unshaved women (probably as a result of minor nicks or cuts caused by the shaving). Also, the itch when the hair grows back is considerable. It should be noted, too, that having somebody go over your pubic area with a razor while you are attempting to keep on top of a contraction, even in early labor, is not fun. It may increase the mother's tension.

Many hospitals are now permitting a "mini-prep," a clipping of the hair instead of shaving, much less uncomfortable.

Enemas, usually given in North American hospitals to women in early labor, create more room in the pelvic cavity and prevent bowel movement during later stages of labor. Many women find this procedure helpful, if unpleasant. Often, however, the mother's body has provided this very service: diarrhea is a common sign of incipient labor, and often continues spontaneously throughout the first stage. Bowel movement itself helps stimulate contractions. If you know

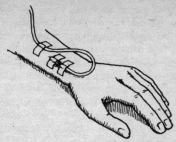

Intravenous (I.V.) drip is used to provide laboring women with glucose or dextrose, to give Pitocin or other labor-stimulating agents, to give Demerol and other analgesics, and to administer blood transfusions.

your bowels are empty, you should tell the appropriate nurse; you may not need an enema.

I.V. (intravenous) procedures have also become routine. Many hospitals automatically attach the I.V. rigging to a woman when she arrives in labor. A vein in the woman's hand (usually) is punctured and a hollow tube is inserted and kept in place. The tube connects to a bottle, which could be used to store an anesthetic or analgesic, labor-stimulating hormones like oxytocin, or blood in case of need for transfusion. The I.V. is used regularly to administer glucose (sugar water) when the attendant(s) thinks the mother needs it to restore energy. This "just-in-case" procedure is useful in a small percentage of labors; for the others it can be a bother. When a woman gets up to go to the bathroom—which is recommended during labor—she must bring with her the metal I.V. stand. The needle in her hand restricts her movement in bed. More than the annoyance of this procedure, the presence of this paraphernalia contributes to making hospital birth seem like a surgical, risky, doctor-determined experience.

It is routine procedure in North American hospitals to not allow the laboring woman to eat or drink, and to use the I.V. glucose as a substitute for sustenance. Food is withheld from the laboring woman in order to reduce gastrointestinal crowding, to give the uterus as much room as possible. Once labor begins, the body shuts down digestive processes to a great extent; so food eaten recently or during labor will have a tendency to remain in the system. The other reason for not allowing women in labor to eat or (usually) drink, except for ice chips, is the contingency that the labor would require general anesthetic. Surgical patients in a hospital are not allowed to eat for at least 12 hours before surgery for the same reason: a person rendered unconscious by a general anesthetic may experience nausea, vomit, and then choke (possibly fatally) on the vomitus, or could take food particles into the lungs, causing aspiration pneumonia.

However, left to nature, women rarely desire heavy food during labor. European hospitals and maternity centers usually offer easily-digested, strengthening liquids, such as broth, sweetened tea, perhaps fruit juice, and maybe light snack food, such as crackers. Surgery under general anesthesia is a less frequent outcome of pregnancy in Europe than here; they do not practice as much plan-for-the-exception medicine as we tend to. U.S. maternity centers usually follow the European lead in this regard.

Forceps

In 1588 the Chamberlen brothers in England invented the obstetrical forceps, a pair of tongs made of metal, which could be inserted into the vagina, applied one to each side of the baby's head, and then pulled, extracting the infant from the birth canal.

The new invention was kept a secret by the inventors, who had an eye for drama and a sense of family pride. When a woman was having the kind of difficult labor which usually ended in mutilation and death of the fetus and severe trauma or even death of the mother, the brothers would arrive with their instrument in a chest, order everyone out of the room, drape and blindfold the woman so that not even she knew what was going on, apply the forceps, and collect their handsome fee. For nearly a century, they refused to part with the secret of their success. When at last they sold the instrument, they tricked the buyer and sold only one half of the forceps. By this time, however, the nature of the mysterious tool had been guessed at, and the *mains de fer* (hands of iron) were secure in their place in what was becoming the surgical specialty of obstetrics.

Midwives of the time, as Adrienne Rich points out in *Of Woman Born*, were outspoken in their opposition to the instrument. Hands of flesh, they said, were appropriate for helping to bring a child into the world; these men with their tools should be called in only as a last resort. The use of forceps as a "quick-delivery trick" was, they believed, wrong and un-natural.

In North America today a different attitude prevails. Dr. Arthur Gorbach, in *Pregnancy, Birth & the Newborn Baby*, states that until the "modern era" forceps were used only for difficult deliveries; but since the early part of this century, "America's obstetricians have come to use forceps for most of their deliveries, even the uncomplicated ones." Estimates of the use of forceps in American hospitals range from 25% to 65% (Canadian figures would be similar). Higher figures come from teaching hospitals. In Holland the figure is around 2%, in England 5%.

Properly applied, forceps do not cause permanent damage to the baby or the mother. Tearing of the mother's vaginal tissue is a possible side-effect. If the application is careless, there is a chance of injuring the baby's head, a remote chance of brain damage to the child.

A baby delivered by forceps will have red bruise marks on her temples or cheeks for a day or two. An uncommon hazard is temporary paralysis of the nerve on the side of the face, occurring mostly in a difficult high- or mid-forceps delivery. Some researchers see a correlation between the unusually tough pulling which occurs in a mid-forceps or high-forceps delivery (quite rare these days) and incidence of cerebral palsy. Mid-forceps and high-forceps refer to how far up the birth canal the instrument must be introduced; low-forceps is the way it is mostly done today, for those last few inches.

Using the forceps can be quite a labor. I have seen it only once, in a film, "The Chicago Maternity Center Story." The obstetrician, Dr. Beatrice Tucker, is attending at a home birth. The baby is in posterior position, and the labor has been long. Dr. Tucker inserts the two sides of the forceps, and then braces herself against the dining room (delivery) table, and really *works* to pull the baby out. I was surprised to see what an arduous task it is. (My friend Jonah, who is 13, was helped out that way too, and his father, who was there, reports the same thing: a surprisingly strenuous pull-and-tug effort is necessary.)

Application of Forceps. Baby is in the usual vertex presentation.

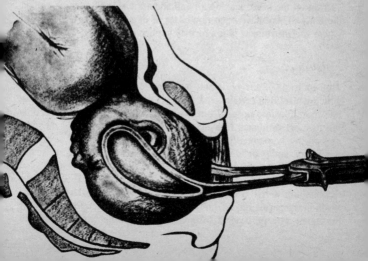

Use of forceps usually entails a generous episiotomy.

The medical reasons for using forceps include: (1) if there is fetal distress, that is, fetal heartbeat goes below 100 beats per minutes or above 160, forceps may be introduced to effect speedy delivery; (2) if the umbilical cord is wrapped around the neck of the baby (which occurs in about 25% of deliveries), or if the cord prolapses, that is, drops into the vaginal canal before the baby does, in which event it could be compressed between the baby and the mother and the oxygen supply would get cut off; (3) for breech presentations, in which the expulsion is more demanding for the mother and often exhausts her; (4) when regional anesthetics remove the mother's ability to push her baby out; and (5) when, for any reason, the second, expulsive stage of labor has in the opinion of the accoucheur gone on too long.

The use of forceps may, on the other hand, be elective. When forceps are necessary to insure the safety of the child and/or the mother, there is, of course, no argument about their use. Indeed, we are all grateful for the lives saved because hands of iron were available to extricate an infant otherwise hopelessly stuck. What an expectant mother and father will want to know is, where there is no anticipated obstetric *need* for forceps delivery, can the woman giving birth "elect" to not have this intervention? This is a matter which should be discussed in advance with whoever will be assisting during the birth.

In some European countries *vacuum extraction* of the fetus—a practice developed in Sweden—is more common than extraction by forceps. In this procedure, a suction cup is applied to the scalp of the descending fetus during the second stage of labor; a machine pulls by suction on the head, leaving a lump about the size of a tennis ball on the baby. There have been rare cases of damage to the baby's head where the instrument is improperly applied.

Episiotomy

This incision of the perineum is a classic example of a technique which is useful in certain situations, yet which, because of its routine incorporation into hospital birth, has become controversial. According to most estimates I have found, the number of births where an episiotomy is *medically* necessary is less than one out of seven. In American and Canadian hopsital births, about six out of seven mothers undergo this procedure. In the Netherlands, 6% to 8% of women have episiotomies; in England, approximately 15% do.

Episiotomy, first described as a surgical procedure in 1870, is a cut made in the perineum, leading away from the vaginal opening toward the anus. The purpose is to enlarge the opening, to facilitate the

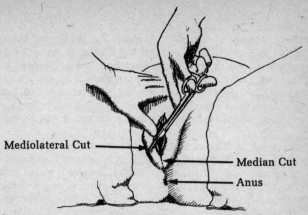

Mediolateral Cut

Median Cut

Anus

Episiotomy. The diagram shows the two possible choices for the cut many women receive to enlarge the birth opening. The incision can prevent tearing.

emergence of the baby. It is neither as horrifying a procedure as many women believe beforehand, nor so insignificant to the woman as most doctors have tended to assume. Indeed, women everywhere express great concern about episiotomy.

To what extent is episiotomy an elective procedure?

English midwife Maggie Myles devotes a section of her *Textbook for Midwives* to "Prevention of Perineal Laceration." She lists the following indications for episiotomy: (1) delay of delivery due to a rigid perineum (that is, the tissue is not stretching sufficiently); (2) disproportion in size between the head of the fetus and the vaginal opening (cephalopelvic disproportion); (3) fetal distress (the episiotomy makes delivery quicker); (4) facilitation in the use of forceps; (5) breech delivery; (6) presence of heart trouble in the mother such that her bearing-down effort would be reduced; (7) a previous tear which would likely re-open; and (8) an effort to save a premature baby the stress of being battered against the perineum.

Another contemporary English midwifery text, by Jean Hallum, approaches the subject of episiotomy this way: "A normal delivery has been described in some detail. Unfortunately at this present age of speed, there is a tendency to encourage midwives to hasten both the second and third stages of labour. The perineum can be incised (episiotomy) but this is seldom necessary in a normal labour. . . . Midwives must know how to perform an episiotomy in an emergency to prevent a severe perineal tear or prolonged pressure of a small foetal head on the perineum.''

Williams Obstetrics, a standard textbook for physicians, treats episiotomy as a given; the question is not whether to do one, but rather when and how to sew it up. In general, the reason given to the hospital-birthing woman (if she hears an explanation) and the justification most often given in standard obstetric texts, is that without the neat perineal incision a tear may occur anyway and it will be jagged, more difficult to repair, and less quick to heal than the episiotomy itself.

Prior to the incision a local anesthetic—usually Xylocaine® (lidocaine), similar to Novacain®—is injected between contractions into the perineal tissue. In one to two minutes the area is numb. The only dangers directly associated with the application of this local anesthetic arise from the possibility that the injection might inadvertently be misdirected—into a blood vessel, for instance, which would case a dangerously high level of the drug to be present in the maternal blood—or from the possibility of accidentally administering too high a dose. Care, of course, must be taken by the midwife or the doctor that the injection not touch the baby.

Episiotomy incisions follow one of two standard patterns; either a median, or mid-line incision, directly toward the anus from the vagina; or a mediolateral oblique cut. The incision itself is made with scissors.

In terms of the woman's comfort, the median is easier to repair and bleeds less, but carries the risk of extension into the anal sphincter, possibly causing debilitating injury. The mediolateral incision, though harder on the woman, allows more room for the baby.

Myles' English midwifery text points out that timing is critical in performing an episiotomy: if the cut is made too early, the perineal tissue is still too thick, and there will be much more bleeding. Further, the baby's head, when it is lodged against the perineum, displaces an important muscle, the *levator ani;* if this displacement has not taken place, that muscle may be damaged by a hasty incision. If the incision is delayed too long, the pelvic floor is overly stretched, the tissues bruised, or the purpose of the episiotomy may be defeated, that is, a tear may have already happened.

Cuts and tears are distinguished as to degree. A third-degree cut, the deep episiotomy, involves skin, mucous membrane, perineal muscles, and the anal sphincter. A first-degree tear, not uncommon without an episiotomy, injures only the skin and the mucous membrane. If the perineal muscles are included, it is considered a second-degree injury. Dr. Gregory White of Chicago, author of *Emergency Childbirth* and pioneer among obstetricians becoming interested in home birth, notes that in 30 years of experience he has never seen a third-degree tear in a natural delivery. To get an injury of that seriousness, he suggests, takes an episiotomy.

The tissues of the vagina soften and become remarkably elastic in the last few weeks of pregnancy. At the time of birth, these tissues are ready to stretch and loosen even more, to permit the passage of the baby. Whereas the opening up of the cervix occurs over a period of hours, the vaginal orifice must do its expansion almost instantly, especially if it is a fast second stage. The need for episiotomy can be avoided if these tissues are allowed time to expand, if the mother is able to pant rather than push and the midwife or doctor is able to ease the head out, massaging the perineum and waiting. Modern obstetrical practice in our tradition almost never emphasizes this possiblity; obstetricians rarely want to take the extra time. They are not taught to give it much consideration. But midwifery has always emphasized allowing nature to take her time, and among midwives it is a matter of pride to have the skill to allow a delivery "over an intact perineum," as they say.

Midwives and obstetricians vary considerably in their attitude toward and performance of episiotomies. Constance Bean describes in *Labor & Delivery* how she watched an obstetrician do a huge, deep cut and asked a nurse afterwards why the cut had been so large. The nurse's only comment was that that doctor was known thereabouts as "the butcher." A matter of personal style.

A Barefoot Doctor's Manual, the standard reference work for paramedicals in Hunan Province, China, describes how birth of the baby's head is managed: "When the head of the baby is exposed [the midwife or physician should] use the right palm, by separating the thumb and the four fingers, to support and protect the perineum." There is no mention of doing any cutting. Massage and support/pressure on the perineum are in fact standard methods for midwives. A lay midwife I spoke to recently says she rarely has to do an episiotomy. She uses hot compresses and perineal pressure, and counts on the woman's being able to "put her brains in her bottom," and really relax to open up. Elizabeth Noble, author of *Essential Exercises for the Childbearing Year*, concurs with this way of managing second-stage labor.

Ways to help prevent the need for episiotomy also include having the mother use a squatting or semi-upright, gravity-enhancing position; and, as Noble points out, if the second stage is *too* rapid, the woman can use a side-lying position and thus bring about a slower, smoother descent.

In *The Cultural Warping of Childbirth*, Doris Haire points to *routine* episiotomy as one factor which illustrates her theme: "It would appear callous indeed for a physician or nurse-midwife to perform an episiotomy without first making an effort to avoid the need for an episiotomy by removing the mother's legs from the stirrups and bringing her up into a semi-sitting position in order to relieve tension on her perineum and enable her to push more effectively.''

So the factors determining whether or not you have an episiotomy may turn out to be (1) time—whether or not you and the doctor or midwife take the time to let the perineum stretch its fullest, and delay the final, gentle pushing until the opening is big enough for the baby to fit through; (2) teamwork—whether or not you and the doctor or midwife have prepared yourselves to try together for a non-episiotomy delivery; and (3) skill—whether the attendant has expertise in knowing how to avoid the cut.

Repair from episiotomy is suturing, sewing; the local anesthetic usually given for the cut suffices for the repair. Recuperation from this procedure is generally only a week or two, although some women are plagued by discomfort for longer. Many women report that the only lasting pain from the whole process of birthing was that ''little cut,'' requiring local anesthetic sprays, repeated sitz-baths, heat lamps, and a temporary shuffle instead of a walk.

Klaus and Kennell, whose concern, as we have seen, is the bonding between parents and newborn, suggest that we consider ''the effects of episiotomy repairs on the comfort, mobility, and ability of the mother to care for her baby.'' The discomfort in recovering from this surgery could upset the ability of some women to relax comfortably in a chair and satisfactorily establish nursing.

Research shows that an uncut perineum springs back to normal with proper exercising better than a cut and sutured one. Moreover, tissue which has been cut and repaired is less stretchable; thus, having once had an episiotomy, it is quite likely that you will have one again in a subsequent birth.

Still, something can be said for the other side. My friend Janet wrote to me regarding my writing this book: ''Remember to include what a woman who had had totally natural childbirth told me a few years ago—that even without anesthetic, the episiotomy was such a glorious relief that she didn't even feel it. Pro and con to that, but there it is. . . .'' Individuals *do* have different tolerances.

Episiotomy is sometimes welcome; controversy, again, concerns the *routine* performance of the procedure in American hospital birth. In this matter, as in many, the line between a procedure which is medically required (or simply routine) and one which is optional or elective is not easy to define. Consequently we, as potential ''patients,'' are given some room to maneuver in. You can in some sense decide for yourself how you feel about such a practice, how much it matters to you from what you know, and set about finding a birth attendant and an institution where you will have some reasonable expectation of arranging such details to your satisfaction.

Induction and stimulation of labor

There are times when an obstetrician decides not to wait for labor to begin spontaneously, but rather to induce it mechanically and/or chemically. Once labor has begun, the same techniques are also used to speed labor up or to stimulate a labor that is lethargic.

Medical reasons for induction of labor are given as: (1) serious disease or condition of the mother, such as diabetes, Rh mis-match, pre-eclampsia; and (2) pronounced postmaturity of the fetus, or clear placental insufficiency. (Sometimes mentioned as a legitimate reason for induction is to accommodate a situation where the mother has a history of delivering very quickly and lives a long way from the hospital; her time for labor thus gets planned in advance.)

The first way to induce or stimulate labor is mechanical. A sharp instrument is introduced into the vagina and pierces the amniotic sac, letting the fluid out. For reasons not fully understood, this procedure, called *amniotomy*, usually sets off uterine contractions within hours. (Spontaneous rupture of membranes has the same effect.) In a case where labor has begun, but seems to be becoming dysfunctional, rupturing of the membranes hastens and tones up uterine contractions.

The second method of induction or stimulation is chemical. The contraction-regulating hormone, *oxytocin*, is administered in its synthetic form, Pitocin® or Syntocinon®. A substance called prostaglandin is being introduced as an alternative to the oxytocins. Prostaglandins, found naturally in semen and menstrual fluid (and elsewhere), stimulate uterine contractility, can reduce blood pressure, and affect the action of some hormones. In *New Miracles of Childbirth* Elliott McCleary reports Dr. Gerald G. Anderson of the medical college of Yale University as saying that prostaglandins seem to be "just as safe" as oxytocin, and are faster. This is not necessarily reassuring.

The method of administering the induction chemical is significant. Induced contractions will vary in their length and strength according to the dose given. The most precise way to administer Pitocin is with the use of an infusion pump. Less precise, but more widely available, is the I.V. drip method. In oral administration (i.e., *buccally*, by mouth) a wafer of Pitocin is put into the mother's mouth to dissolve gradually; this is not a very precise method. Intramuscular injection of Pitocin is the least controllable of all.

Sometimes both induction methods, mechanical and chemical, are used together.

Dr. Roberto Caldeyro-Barcia (president of the International Federation of Gynecologists and Obstetricians) has studied the effects of labor induction on the baby, particularly mechanical induction by the rupturing of the membranes. He has found that once the membranes are ruptured, the baby's head has no cushion, and great misalignment and deformation of the fetal skull may take place from being pounded unprotected against the cervix; with this there is the increase in the possibility of brain damage.

Chemical induction of labor requires close supervision. The actual effects of the procedure on any individual labor are far from predictable, no matter how closely the administering of the drug is watched. The most noticeable result of Pitocin-induction is the change in quality of uterine contractions. Varying according to the amount of Pitocin, the method of administering, and the tolerance of the individual's system, these contractions are often longer, more violent and painful, than noninduced contractions, and they tend to lack the characteristic wavelike rhythm of building up and dropping off. Rest periods between these contractions are shorter.

One woman I know had planned a medication-free, Lamaze-style delivery. More than 48 hours after her waters broke (in an Italian restaurant), contractions had not yet begun. Her doctor told her to check in at the hospital, which she did, with her husband, Lamaze kit in hand. After two hours in the labor room and no contractions yet, Pitocin was administered. The dosage must have been large; contractions came fast and hard. Early labor had been by-passed altogether and the contractions were suddenly overwhelming. There had been no building-up to them, no time to develop a rhythm of breathing or a feel for the waves. All the Lamaze training for this event became at once useless. The husband was asked to leave, an anesthetic was administered, and in less than three hours the mother, a primapara, was delivered of her baby (who, as it turned out, was just fine).

From the start, then, the woman whose labor is chemically induced has a more difficult task to overcome and has an increased likelihood of wanting or needing other drugs and procedures.

Induction is harder on the baby, too. Because of the more violent uterine activity, the baby gets pounded more forcefully against the opening cervix and must endure a correspondingly greater interruption in oxygen supply. Distress and anoxia are not uncommon in induced labors; one estimate says that distress occurs two times more often in induced babies than in noninduced.

Another potential danger from labor induction is abruptio placenta; if the uterus contracts too vigorously under Pitocin stimulation, the placenta may become dislodged from the uterine lining. Induction can also result in excessive tension, spasm, and possible rupture of the uterus, and excessive bleeding postpartum. Another hazard of induction is noted in *Redbook* magazine (August, 1974). A report, based on a study of 1000 induced births and 1000 noninduced births, concluded that 10% of the *premature* births in our country are due to "elective" inductions and "elective" Caesarean sections. That is, estimates of fetal maturity had been in error, resulting in the births of children who otherwise would not have had to contend with the stress and dangers of prematurity.

With these sobering facts in mind, it becomes hard to justify the degree of permissiveness toward (even encouragement of) these procedures among American and Canadian and even British doctors and hospitals. Yet there is an overall induction rate of 10%. In one month in 1975, in a Chicago hospital, 55% of all deliveries were oxytocin-induced. While Dr. Caldeyro-Barcia estimates that only 3% of births need this kind of stimulation, 90% of inductions are performed on otherwise normal labors.

The medical reasons for induction of labor have been stated. It should be noted, too, that speed, or expediency, is another kind of reason for inducing and stimulating labor. There seems to be an attitude (alarmingly prevalent in the U.S.) that labor should always be hustled along. This is practical, of course, from the point of view of the overworked obstetrician and the understaffed hospital. It is a kind of convenience factor. It is an attempt to regularize the hours which a birth attendant works. Some mothers, too, *want* to have labor induced, want to plan for the time when the birth will occur.

Yet convenience may be in conflict with the best interests of both mother and child. Nurse-midwife Barbara Brennan, in her *Complete Book of Midwifery,* remarks that "Midwives *never* induce labor for our own convenience or for our patients', either." Dr. Frederic Ettner, a Chicago-based obstetrician and contributor to NAPSAC's *Safe Alternatives in Childbirth,* characterizes appropriate medical induction as limited to those situations "in which continuation of pregnancy would present an absolute threat to the life or well-being of the mother or her child." Considering the problems and hazards of induction, this may turn out to be the best criterion.

Fetal heart monitor

A safe fetal heart rate is considered to be between 120 and 160 beats per minute. Concern arises when the rate goes above 160 or below about 110, indicating distress. The more we know about the effects of oxygen deprivation of the brain, the more concerned we are about insuring that the unborn receives his due of oxygen; it is the heartbeat that reports to us how sturdy that small heart actually is.

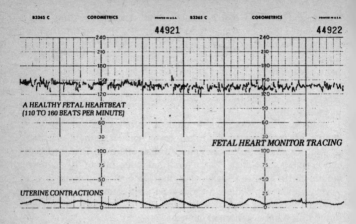

A HEALTHY FETAL HEARTBEAT
(110 TO 160 BEATS PER MINUTE)

FETAL HEART MONITOR TRACING

UTERINE CONTRACTIONS

The fetal heart monitor (of which there are now many varieties) is a relatively new device now in use in many hospitals and maternity centers in this country. Designed in the late 1950s in California by Dr. Edwin Hon, it electronically records fetal heartbeat. Its purpose is to detect complications and abnormalities in the heartbeat of the unborn. The fetal heart monitor (fhm) consists of a stereo-size machine with straps which are attached by jelly/glue to the woman's abdomen in two places: the upper one records uterine contractions, the lower one records the heartbeat of the fetus. A specialist must monitor this procedure frequently. Accuracy of interpretation is a problem, as the external leads may pick up vibrations from other sources, such as the mother's intestines. In order to be quite accurate, the *internal* monitoring system of the machine may be put to use. In this procedure, electrodes are screwed to the scalp of the fetus after the cervix is partly opened up; these are attached by a clip or screw to a plastic tube, or catheter, which has been passed up the vagina, and from there to the machine.

Though the traditional method of monitoring fetal heartbeat (using a special stethoscope) is quite adequate in normal birth, the fetal heart monitor is a valuable addition to high-risk, induced, and problem labors. It can detect a pattern of trouble which, if read by experienced technicians, will alert the obstetrical team to the need to interfere, probably with a Caesarean section. Statistics show that infant mortality rates have declined where the monitor is used; however, as Suzanne Arms points out, this may be as much due to the added care which use of a monitor entails as to the machine itself.

The fetal heart monitor is also used in what is called a "stress test," a way of determining the condition of the baby who is postmature or who may be in distress for other reasons. A small amount of Pitocin is administered to the woman, the fhm is attached (external leads), and the fetal heart rate is interpreted. This is a way of asking the baby how he is. If the baby's heart beat accelerates as a result of the Pitocin-induced contractions, he is probably not in trouble. If, on the other hand, the heartbeat slows down, the condition of the baby is of concern, and a decision may be made to do a Caesarean section.

Predictably, rates of Caesarean section usually rise when a monitor is introduced into a hospital or maternity center. One obstetrician to whom Arms spoke declared that even a 25% chance of accuracy in an fhm reading is sufficient for him to immediately decide to do a C-section. Caesarean rates in facilities where the device has been in use for a while, however, return to a more normal level (see the next section for some interpretations of what is a "normal" level of Caesarean).

Proponents of this device claim with electronic monitoring of most labors, Caesarean sections are now performed more where they really are needed and less where they really aren't. They also remind us that induced and stimulated labors require careful monitoring because the force of induced contractions is so unpredictable and possibly deadly. The fetal heart monitor, therefore, they say, may be saving some mothers and babies a lot of stress by indicating when the Pitocin drip needs to be decreased.

There are drawbacks. To be valuable as a predictor, the machine requires constant, educated surveillance of its output. The woman must remain pretty much supine, a position well known to put pressure on her blood supply to the fetus and to be generally uncomfortable for her. For internal monitoring, rupture of the membranes of the amniotic sac is necessary; this increases the chance for infection and excessive bleeding, and may lead to the need for further intervention. And the internal electrodes do get clipped or screwed to the baby's head.

Some women are more uncomfortable strapped to a machine than others. *Our Bodies, Ourselves,* which provides excellent coverage of this and other obstetric devices and procedures, reports these two contrasting experiences: "I had a belt around my abdomen to monitor my contractions and a monitor inserted into my vagina attached to my baby's head to monitor her heartbeat. The belt kept slipping off and felt very uncomfortable. I felt like I couldn't move and was annoyed by that restriction." And: "I felt very reassured by the monitor. I could see when my contractions began and ended, and I could see my baby's heart beating. I had an epidural so I didn't feel anything. It was nice to be able to know that everything was proceeding normally, since I couldn't feel what was happening.''

Many couples find it a novel, pleasantly distracting experience to be able to trace the contractions as they blip across the paper in the machine. As with the woman quoted above, some are reassured by the evidence of the heartbeat of the baby in such scientific form.

Because of the cost of these machines (approximately $5000 at present), most facilities do not come close to being able to monitor every woman in labor. One estimate suggests that 10% of labors are monitored at this time. But not every laboring woman needs to be monitored. At Booth Maternity Center in Philadelphia, there are two monitors, so a woman whose labor is atypical or showing signs of trouble will be the one most consistently hooked up. At Booth, they like to monitor every labor for a little while.

A Dutch obstetrician reported to Suzanne Arms that the machines were put away when it was realized that the mothers were receiving much less personal attention since the coming of the monitors; henceforth, they were to be used only in cases of genuine medical need.

When Dr. Caldeyro-Barcia, who, with Dr. Hon, has been a pioneer in interpretation of tracing equipment, was questioned about the need for monitoring all laboring women and the possibility of funding for such an enterprise, he replied by offering the opinion that ''more lives could be saved by spending this money to buy food for the world's pregnant women than to monitor them.''

The decision-making process during labor and delivery is sometimes the drama of split-seconds and sudden surgery; sometimes it is in watching a record of the heartbeat over many hours, how the rate hovers on the border between safety and distress. The story of the fetal heart monitor is not just in how it feels to wear one, or even in a statistical review of the Caesarean-section rate in relation to fhm use. The broadest concern is in how great a role such a machine will be designated to carry in decision-making during the course of labor. If an institution is to consult the fhm as an advisor regarding fetal health during labor, benefit comes by using the device only with the highest degree of precision, by accurately learning the language of this new technology.

SURGERY: CAESAREAN SECTION

Margaret Mead said (on the N.E.T. production ''Giving Birth''): ''I think it is sheer ideology, you know, to insist that you should never use drugs, or you should always use drugs. All of the complicated kinds of equipment that we have developed for childbirth have been developed with some kind of reason originally. There *are* cases where childbirth *is* surgery. And this of course is the question of a Caesarean. This is surgery, it is good surgery, it saves the baby who might otherwise have died.'' Indeed, we are grateful to the experimentally-inclined early barber-surgeons who turned to obstetrics, to the hundreds of practitioners, frantic husbands, midwives, and doctors who perfected the technique we call Caesarean section, childbirth by surgery.

Whether it be fact or fancy that the Roman Julius was delivered in this manner, whether the name derives from the Latin verb *caedere*, ''to cut,'' we do know that Caesarean sections have been performed for centuries. In the early days, that is, until around the mid-eighteenth century, the results were predictably dire, certain death for the mother and questionable survival for the infant.

In 1739 an Irish midwife, Mary Donally, took out a razor, cut open the abdomen of a woman who had been laboring for 12 days, removed the dead child, and sewed up the lady with silk. A month later, the woman could walk a mile. Yet maternal survival of this operation at that time was close to zero.

Now nearly one of five women who enter a hospital in many locales in North America (especially in well-endowed, high-risk, teaching facilities) will emerge postoperative, having given birth under the knife. Although countless lives have been saved in this way, the procedure is under question. Why is the Caesarean rate in this country and Canada approaching 25%, higher than anywhere in the world? Holland, regarded by Arms as the ''Caretaker of Normal Birth,'' has a Caesarean section rate of about 4%.

In surgical childbirth, the obstetrcian cuts through the layers of the abdomen, into the uterus, and lifts the baby out. The incision is often vertical (the classical C-section technique). When emergency conditions are not present—when, that is, the surgery is elective or pre-planned—the surgeon may choose to cut through the uterus lower down, in a lateral direction, where the uterus is thicker and less likely to rupture. This surgery is traditionally done under general anesthetic. But recently there has been a rise in the use of regional (spinal) anesthetic for Caesareans; this allows the mother to see her infant immediately and avoids the dangers of (and recuperation from) a general anesthetic. In either case it is major abdominal surgery, requiring intensive postoperative care.

Reasons for using this method of childbirth include: cepahlo-pelvic disproportion (the baby's head is larger than the mother's pelvis can accommodate); severe diabetes; toxemia-pre-eclampsia in the mother;

abruption of placenta, placenta previa, or cord prolapse; difficult breech presentation; previous C-section. Modern obstetrics is adding to the list: prolonged labor (open to the obstetrician's interpretation); uterine inertia (constractions are not accomplishing dilatation); and severe fetal distress.

Sectioning of breech babies is now performed routinely on women experiencing a first pregnancy, and is highly likely with multiparae. Most hospital personnel haven't seen a vaginal delivery of a breech baby in years. The last time my obstetrician did one, he said, it was like Grand Central Station, as everyone came running to watch. There is now emerging a generation of doctors to whom this art is a lost one. The baby, argues modern obstetrics, must endure a dangerous level of stress in its intricate vaginal passage when the buttocks or feet are presenting; the risk is not worth it.

My friend Betsy, a primapara in her early thirties, described her Caesarean experience to me.

As instructed by her obstetrician, Betsy went to the hospital (in Ontario) when her waters broke; some 20 hours later, labor finally seemed to be establishing itself. Betsy's blood-sugar level was low during the next 10 hours of active labor. She was given simple I.V. glucose, which acted to increase her contractions in both duration and intensity. For the last three or four hours, Betsy reports, "I had quite strong contractions lasting about a minute until building to a plateau, another minute with an intense desire to push, another minute of contraction, and then about a thirty-second pause before the set started again. Throughout all of this, I managed to dilate only 3 centimeters, which was a bit depressing. It was also apparent that the labor was hardly following the books, and nurses mentioned to us (her husband Tom was with her) that we should be prepared for some kind of intervention. . . . As soon as my obstetrician examined me, he said that a section would be necessary, because of the angle of Catherine's head . . . apparently she was head-down, in posterior position, but with her forehead rather than her crown proceeding first, and being hung up on the pubic bone. . . . I was prepped for surgery quickly, and in half an hour was in the operating room. Tom was not allowed to accompany me.

"Caesarean delivery under local anesthetic was definitely weird and somewhat uncomfortable, but presumably no more so than vaginal delivery. The obstetrician apparently believed he was explaining things to me as he went along, but the drainage tube passed by my ear and made his explanations inaudible. The nurse in surgery who stood near my head and held my hand was a great help and support. And probably it was just as well that a surgical drape obscured my view of the operation. After the delivery, I was allowed to touch but not hold (being covered with tubes) Catherine.

"I went to surgical recovery for an hour—a most unpleasant room—and then to the maternity ward. With quite a bit of persuasion, Tom and I managed to have Catherine brought to us from the intensive care nursery where she had automatically been shipped because of the section delivery, even though she had not had any anesthetics. We were then allowed to be together, alone, for about an hour. A precious, wonderful time."

Under what circumstances should a Caesarean be performed? Drs. Greenhill and Friedman, in *Biological Principles and Modern Practice of Obstetrics,* posit the following criterion: "It is unfortunate that there are practitioners who inappropriately resort to caesarean section whenever they are confronted with a difficult obstetric situation or a medical or surgical problem in an obstetric patient. Although some of these operations are clearly justified, many are not. Clinicians are admonished to understand that delivery by Caesarean section must be reserved only for those patients in whom vaginal delivery cannot be accomplished without seriously jeopardizing fetal or maternal life and health." In Besty's case, the extreme duration of her labor in combination with the irregularity of Catherine's presentation clearly justified the surgical intervention.

Women who have had a Caesarean section have many reactions. Some feel cheated, some feel guilty, many feel overwhelmingly grateful to have survived and to have a healthy child. All are glad for whatever relevant information they had stored away or were given beforehand; knowing what was going on definitely reduced their panic and their anxiety. It is usually true, but not always, that once you have had a Caesarean, all subsequent deliveries will have to follow suit.

Recovery, settling into feeding, re-establishing of gastrointestinal routines, these are all unique for C-section mothers.

A planned Caesarean is much less traumatic, of course, than an emergency one. But in either case, being able to share your feelings about the birth, especially with other Caesarean parents, is important. There is at least one organization devoted to this concern; it is located in the Boston area, and is called C/Sec (address given as c/o Melissa Foley, 15 Maynard Road, Dedham, Massachusetts 02026). Local chapters of ICEA would be another source of information about such groups. (See also Chapter 6.)

4

Midwives
and Other Friends

Childbirth throughout human history, around the world and across the centuries, reveals one pattern consistently: women in labor are attended by someone, most of all by a woman or women whose calling it is to be there. She is what our English ancestors called the midwife, a word meaning *with woman*. In the Latin language she is, similarly, *cum-mater*, and in Spanish and Portuguese *comadre*. Among the ancient Jews she was known as the "wise woman," a characterization of almost universal prevalance that is rendered precisely in the modern German *weise frau* and French *sage-femme*.

The midwife has always been a figure of controversy, representing power and control in the miraculous bringing forth of life itself. Her work has served humankind as a metaphor even where and when that work in its concrete form was restricted or outlawed. Socrates claimed that his mission in life was that of a midwife, to deliver the "new man," to aid in bringing forth the enlightened one. Whether it is read metaphorically or literally, the following excerpt from Plato's dialogue of *Theatetus* stresses the midwife's aged wisdom and power over life:

> SOCRATES: Bear in mind the whole business of midwives, and then you will see my meaning better:—no woman, as you are probably aware, who is still able to conceive and bear, attends other women, but only those who are past bearing.
>
> THEATETUS: Yes, I know.
>
> SOCRATES: The reason of this is said to be that Artemis—the goddess of childbirth—is not mother, and she honors those who are like herself; but she could not allow the barren to be midwives, because human nature cannot know the mystery of an art without experience; and therefore she assigned this office to those who are too old to bear.
>
> THEATETUS: I dare say.
>
> SOCRATES: And I dare say too, or rather I am absolutely certain that the midwives know better than others who is pregnant and who is not?

THEATETUS: Very true.

SOCRATES: And by the use of potions and incantations they are able to arouse the pangs and soothe them at will; they can make those bear who have difficulty in bearing, and if they think fit they can smother the embryo in the womb.

THEATETUS: They can.

Imbued with such powers, it is no wonder that the midwife in history has been a central figure in a drama of medicine, politics, religion, and sexuality. She was condemned as a witch and burned at the stake in medieval Europe. By the beginning of the 16th century, the midwife was eclipsed by the power of the doctor and his techniques. In 1591, a Scottish midwife, Agnes Simpson, was burned to death for attempting to relieve a woman's birth pains with opium. In America, she has been indicted for impudence and ignorance, and has at times seemed to disappear from view. But this wise-woman, this neighbor lady, has never really left the side of the woman in labor—brewing herbal teas, listening to the fetal heartbeat, patiently waiting for nature to follow its course, perhaps dancing and wailing around the laboring one, leaving an axe by the bed with the blade up to cut the pain, or in some places opening the windows and setting horses free from the stable to loosen the labor.

In Puerto Rico, in Yugoslavia, among the Indians of the northwest coast, wherever she finds herself working, it is to her that women bring their family concerns, their problems with sex, their need for abortion, the pain in their groin. She is an archetype, often a goddess; cultures need her just as they need the priest or shaman.

Are we, in fact, so different today?

Worldwide, 80% of newborns are caught by midwives. Although the United States is the only country that has ever actually outlawed midwifery, there is now, in the 1970s, a resurgence of interest in the midwifely fashion of maternity care. Increasing numbers of people are beginning to want to wake up from the medicated helplessness so often typical of delivering in American hospitals. Couples are beginning to want to participate in the birth process as designed by nature, to want protection from unnecessary interference, and to appreciate concern for the whole family as a new life makes its entrance. It is the combination of these qualities which the midwife has to offer.

Western Europe has often been for us a model in this. Colonists brought British midwifery across the Atlantic with them: rural midwifery in the South received a boost from the importation of English, Irish, and Scottish midwives in the late 1920s to Kentucky. The Netherlands, Denmark, and England are among those countries with strong midwifery traditions instituted at the state level with

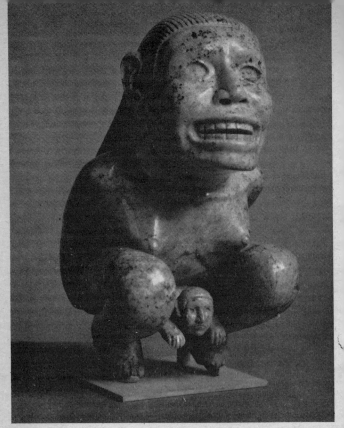

May I introduce Tlazolteotl? She is Aztec; the women who kept her near were Indians in central Mexico some 800 years ago. Her other name is Teteoinnam, patron of midwives, guardian of women in birth. They say she is perpetually giving birth to the Sun God. I have been given a clay version of her, pale sand color, less polished than the Tlazolteotl in this photograph. In the corner of my study she squats, grimacing in the wonderment and strain of her birth throes—a comfort to my labors.

education and licensing, beginning a hundred years ago or more. Indeed, infant and maternal mortality statistics are noticeably better in those countries than here.

Besides the European and other foreign midwives, some 12,000 of whom are estimated to be practicing and studying here now, North America is relying on the services of midwives of many other kinds, from many backgrounds. Some 5000 granny midwives were still practicing in 1973, mostly in the South and West. Birth centers and alternative health clinics, especially in California, have uncovered and created lay midwives to aid the many couples who are choosing not to do business with hospitals; virtually every region of the U.S. has lay midwives practicing independently, however far under cover they must go. The Farm in Tennessee, communal home of some 1100 people and progenitor of several other communities like it around the country, has given birth to its own brand of midwifery and offers this service free to anyone who wants it. And as of 1976, some 1800 Certified Nurse-Midwives were in practice, at hospitals and maternity centers throughout the country, as official partners with doctors on the obstetrical team.

We have of course other help and company in our laboring. It was the court of Louis XIV of France which decided that the male doctor would be the appropriate accoucheur, or attendant at birth. With that, a new medical specialty was born. Obstetricians, 97% of whom are male, still "deliver" at the vast majority of births in our culture. But the role of the obstetrician is now undergoing new definition, approaching more closely—when midwives are in attendance—the original sense of the Latin *obstare,* "to stand by." Nurses who practice in hospitals and nurses who do public health work also figure on the obstetrical team. And, in the last 15 years or so, maternity care has seen another big change: the labor and delivery room doors have in many facilities been opened to allow the father to enter, to observe, and, indeed, to *collaborate* in the event.

Within this expanding range of possibilities, we can exert our freedom of choice: we, as expectant parents, are consumers of vastly important, often expensive help, and we do ourselves a disservice if we do not investigate available alternatives in birth attendance. In this chapter we will look at some vignettes of midwifery from colonial through contemporary times, and then look to the idea of choice as it embraces not only the midwife, but the father, the physician, and other providers as well.

LAY MIDWIFERY IN AMERICA

The first midwives in our continent were, of course, Native Americans. Each tribe developed its practices of birthing; the midwives were almost always female blood relatives to the laboring woman. Medicine men, shamans, and tribal magicians traditionally had their role in producing spells for cases of difficult labor. Tribal midwifery is a lore unto itself, from which we have learned perhaps far too little. David Meltzer's anthology *Birth* includes, among its collection of legends, celebrations, customs, and tales about childbirth from around the globe, a few original texts from some of the early American tribes.

When the colonists arrived on these shores in the 17th century, they brought the British tradition of obstetrics with them. A story from that time will give a taste of early American midwifery.

Colonial America: Anne Hutchinson

At a time when middle-class women's work in life was to manage daily cares so that the husband could be free for his meditations on divinity, Anne Hutchinson upset the social order. When she and her husband William arrived in Boston in 1634, their house became at once a center for religious debate. It was not long before Anne, a midwife, extended her activities by leading classlike discussions on theological matters, questioning the exclusion of women from what was referred to as the "priesthood of all believers."

Thus, having intimate power in the realm of childbirth (i.e., sexuality, especially in the eyes of the Church), and also possessing the intelligence and spirit to challenge male religious doctrine, Anne Hutchinson was a formidable threat.

Her opponent, Massachusetts Governor Winthrop, was appalled by her, though fascinated as well. He named her Jezebel, a direct Satanic threat to New England, and described her as one ". . .of a nimble wit and active spirit, and a very voluble tongue, more bold than a man." Anne Hutchinson was condemned, sentenced, and banished from Massachusetts.

Although it came with the British Empire, the art of midwifery, which had spiritual components and theological ramifications, had no welcome beginning among the Anglo-Saxon Americans. For with it came a tradition of British medicine supported by a powerful, anti-feminist Church which held that any attempt to alleviate women's suffering in childbirth was contrary to God's law. For Anne Hutchinson as for countless, unnamed others, this meant that fear, ignorance, and dogma among the male supremacists would inevitably lead to the equation of midwifery with witchcraft.

Rural America: the grannies and the Frontier Nursing Service

In the rural areas of the West and South, in the early part of this century, flourished a special breed of American midwife, the granny or neighbor lady.

Some of these rural women had training, some did not. Their practice grew from the needs of their people, isolated from medical care. They counseled on rest and eating before and after birth; they taught basic baby care; they knew herbs; and they had their superstitions. (Postpartum orders: "Eat anything y'want except kraut and pickled beans, and stay in th'bed for ten days.")

The granny would stay a week or so after the birth. Payment was whatever the family could afford—chickens, a twist of tobacco, day work. Mothers often named a girl child after a favorite granny.

Mrs. Andy Webb, a granny midwife from Georgia, defines the work of herself and her peers (her story is told by Karen Cox in a chapter from *Foxfire* 2 entitled "Midwives and Granny Women"): "I had no teachin' at all, and I *know* it'uz better then because they ain't near as many women were dyin' then as they is now. They was took better care of. I can't read, nor I can't write. What I've got, God gave it t'me. And I'm proud of it, and I've saved many a life. What God gives y'is right. I never lost a patient because I had th'Lord with me, and I was willin' and ready t'do all I could t'save th'lives."

Medically, of course, the grannies were ill-equipped. Realizing that their province was only the normal birth, they arranged for women to be examined whenever possible by a doctor. But for many families, these granny women were the *only* medical care available, and in their heyday, the 1920s and 1930s, they touched thousands of lives. Yet as obstetrical care spread and became hospital-centered in this country, it condemned the granny as ignorant and unclean.

The art of the rural granny midwife in our history is a mixture of community service, strong faith, the teachings of experience, and stubborn devotion. No one of their constituents doubted their skill or hesitated to consult them; whole communities relied on these women. While becoming increasingly scarce in numbers, there are still some grannies around.

Rural midwifery received a momentous boost in 1925, when a remote corner of southeastern Kentucky became the site for a successful experiment in health care.

Mary Breckinridge, a public-health nurse born in Kentucky and trained in England in midwifery, set up the Frontier Nursing Service (FNS) in the most untamed locale she could find, reasoning that a nursing service which could make it there could make it anywhere.

And so it did, in simple rustic buildings, to and from which the mountain people would travel on horseback. During the 1930s the Frontier Nursing Service offered training in nurse-midwifery, and in 1939 the FNS established its own school for midwives. This continues today as the Frontier School of Midwifery and Family Nursing, affiliated with the University of Kentucky.

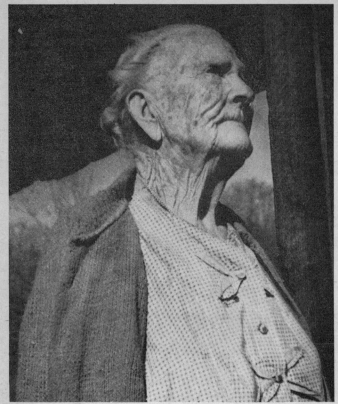

Mrs. Andy Webb, granny midwife from Georgia.

In more than 50 years of rural midwifery, the Kentucky facility has a record to be proud of: the infant mortality rate there is about 6 per 1000 live births, considerably lower than the 10 per 1000 which the American College of Obstetrics and Gynecology has for its goal in the coming decade.

Lay midwifery today: independent midwives and The Farm

Lay midwives have probably always existed in all regions of our continent, practicing quietly, going to homes, often in partnership with a sympathetic doctor. Since the late 1960s, a number of intelligent, outspoken, concerned young women have begun to choose and to visibly change the lay-midwife profession. In parts of California this movement has been especially active.

Nancy Mills, speaking of the lay midwife in *Safe Alternatives in Childbirth* (NAPSAC), tells how she got started: "The way I became involved in midwifery some years after I had my first two children was very accidental. I was actually walking down the road one afternoon (1970) along the river and stopped in to see a friend. This friend happened to be in labor." The friend, it turned out, refused to go to the hospital: ". . . she said, 'No, I won't go. I had my last baby there and it was horrible and I'm going to stay home.' Well, not knowing a thing about it, I was a little concerned. I was a little worried but I stuck around and helped her husband who was having a pretty hard time of it and we delivered the baby. It was really a beautiful experience for me."

After that, word got around in her part of Northern California that Nancy had had experience at births, and the demand for her services began to grow. As of May, 1977, she had helped deliver over 500 babies. Her work now includes research on home birth in California and, with a midwife from Ireland, the establishment of a free maternity clinic.

Though her work grew directly out of a disaffection for hospital birth felt by mostly counterculture couples, Mills emphasizes the need for midwives to be able to understand established medicine: "I've realized that there is a time and place for the hospital, and we need them, and we need to establish a relationship with them where they can respect us and we can respect them."

Another California midwife, Raven Lang, is the author of *Birth Book* and of an obstetrical work for midwives (in progress). She was one of the founders of the controversial Santa Cruz Birth Center in 1971, and of the Vancouver (British Columbia) Birth Center. The Santa Cruz Birth Center offered prenatal care and oversaw home births from 1971 to 1974. Then authorities, using a stooge, stepped in and arrested three midwives for practicing medicine without a license. (I'm reminded of the witch-hunting text *Malleus Maleficarum*, 1484 A.D., popular in Europe for three centuries: "If a woman dare to cure without having studied she is a witch and must die.")

Lay healers, practitioners of peoples' medicine, have always run afoul of "legitimate" medicine. (Ehrenreich and English, my source for the witch-hunting quotation, present a valuable account of this struggle in their booklet *Witches, Midwives, and Nurses*.) Lay midwives are rarely permitted by law to practice fully, that is, to deliver babies as well as provide prenatal care, postnatal care, and labor support. States vary in their laws (and in their enforcement of them); because of the laws, lay midwives must be careful, advertise only by word of mouth, try not to be so visible as to attract trouble, but to be visible enough so that people know they are there. The issue, when legal trouble occurs, is that of practicing medicine without a license.

The closest I've seen to a tribal form of midwifery is the midwifery practiced at The Farm in Summertown, Tennessee.

The Farm was born when a caravan of buses containing 200 or more seekers left San Francisco in 1971 and headed east. Stephen Gaskin, former English professor at San Francisco State College, was and is their leader. They settled on 1700 acres of Tennessee and now they number more than 1100.

Farm midwifery began on the Caravan itself, with Stephen as the first midwife. By the time the group had settled in Tennessee, Ina May and Margaret had become midwives and were beginning to formulate the attitudes which in 1974 were published as *Spiritual Midwifery*, the Farm's own manual. Pamela, one of the women who gave birth en route, tells in the book how she came to be a midwife: "After we settled onto our farm in Tennessee, Ina May was having more and more babies to deliver. She asked me if I could help out by setting up a small first aid station and if I could help her and Margaret with some birthings. It was just what I wanted to do."

I visited the Farm in late February, 1977.

The sunny treatment room at the Farm's Clinic was comfortable and tidy. Over the desk were photographs of the two Guatemalan midwives with whom the Farm midwives have been working in Central America. Pamela explained to me how the midwives run the Clinic (they oversee *all* medical treatment) and work with the pregnant women and deliver the babies. Dr. Williams from the nearby town is their friend, mentor, and backup. There are eight or nine midwives now on the Tennessee Farm, one or two more in Guatemala and/or on other farms. Although they are young (mostly in their twenties), these women have experience. As a group, the midwives function like a religious council to the Farm; their advice and their judgment are highly respected.

I asked one woman I met what kind of work she does on the Farm—everyone does some sort of job—and then asked her if she had ever thought she might like to be a midwife. She explained to me that midwifery isn't a job like the other jobs, where you decide you might like to try it. It happens differently with the midwifing (and with the school-teaching, too). You might first be asked to assist at a birthing, and then gradually take on more and more of the work in a period of careful apprenticeship. It is a calling.

About 600 babies have been born at the Farm, not all of them to

Farm dwellers. There is an open offer: "Don't have an abortion. You can come to the Farm and we'll deliver your baby and take care of it, and if you ever decide you want it back, you can have it"—which, to the available level of housing and Clinic help, they will do.

Their caring is reflected also in the way the Farm midwives speak about their work; it is in the very title of their book. Leslie reminded me: "A midwife handles life and death karma. She is a guide for other people's energy. To be a real midwife, it is necessary to be spiritual. Compassion has to be a way of life for her. The midwife must be able to consider someone else's viewpoint, and in her daily life take care of those around her."

NURSE-MIDWIFERY

Midwifery's youngest branch has developed from within the medical profession in the last four or five decades. Nurse-midwifery was officially recognized in 1971 by the professional organization of the medical/obstetrical community, the American College of Obstetricians and Gynecologists (ACOG). The nurse-midwife, stated ACOG, "may assume complete care and management of uncomplicated maternity patients while serving as a member of an obstetrics team."

Nurse-midwifery training entails a course of study of one to two years after the nursing degree. During her training a nurse-midwife will attend at perhaps 150 deliveries and concentrate as well on other areas of traditional midwife work: prenatal health of mother and baby, postpartum adjustment of the new family.

There are some 24 programs in nurse-midwifery now in the United States. As of early 1979, approximately 2000 Certified Nurse-Midwives (CNMs) were practicing.

Practicing in medicine means becoming "certified," and this entails licensing. For nurse-midwives as for lay midwives, state law and the interpretation of it determine the conditions of their practice, and this varies from state to state. As of the summer of 1976, three states still had what the *Journal of Nurse-Midwifery* refers to as "restrictive interpretation of laws"—Michigan, Kansas, and Wisconsin. Most other states, according to the *Journal,* specify conditions under which nurse-midwives may practice. The Summer, 1976, issue of the *Journal,* a special issue on "Legislation and Nurse-Midwifery Practice in the U.S.A.," lists the laws state by state; most states listed agencies where nurse-midwives are employed for full clinical practice.

But usually a nurse-midwife does not practice independently. You may find her on the staff of a clinic, health center, maternity center, or, since 1964, a hospital. Thus she is always a member of a health-care team. And that facet of obstetrical care in which the CNM specializes relates more to the midwifery tradition than to the medical one. Here we will look at the various kinds of work and working situations of a few Certified Nurse-Midwives.

Jean Brown is a CNM at Penn-Urban Health Maintenance Program, a Philadelphia out-patient clinic, where she serves on a team with a gynecologist/obstetrician, Dr. Cynthia Cooke. Jean delivers no babies (the hospital affiliated with this clinic does not permit CNMs to deliver), but does a great amount of basic office gynecology and is responsible for about half the prenatal care, including arranging for each client to see the staff pediatrician around the seventh month of pregnancy. Dr. Cooke delivers babies, does surgery, shares the prenatal care, and has some special projects, such as working with Women Organized Against Rape.

Interestingly, my own quite automatic reference to Jean Brown as *Jean* (although I do not know her) and to Cynthia Cooke as *Dr.* Cooke (even though I have spoken to her) may raise a basic question: what is the team like that contains one professional and one middle-level practitioner? *how* do they divide the work?

Down the middle and according to specialized areas of interest, it turns out. These are salaried medical-care providers with a sensible division of work-load; they have specific, complementary skills in the large area known as obstetrics. For the professional M.D., who (compared with the middle-level CNM) spent two-to-three times as long in school and who has at least twice the overall backup responsibility as the other, the salary is about double. That is the way this kind of arrangement may work. And it seems to work well. There are gynecology patients at Penn-Urb who never see Dr. Cooke; none of the hospitalized patients, on the other hand, would see Jean Brown. Division of labor in the case of this clinic makes a good team.

Barbara Brennan, whose definition of professional midwifery was cited in the introductory section of this chapter, was the first CNM to practice at a hospital. Since 1964, she has been on the staff at Roosevelt Hospital in New York, attending deliveries and teaching medical students and midwifery students (there are now five CNMs on the staff). Her recent publication (with Joan Heilman) of *The Complete Book of Midwifery,* though perhaps too enthusiastically titled, describes well the work of the present-day nurse-midwife who chooses to practice in a big-city hospital.

"Professional midwives," explains Brennan, "look at pregnancy and childbirth as a normal process, something a woman's body is designed to do and can do by itself 9 times out of 10—by giving the

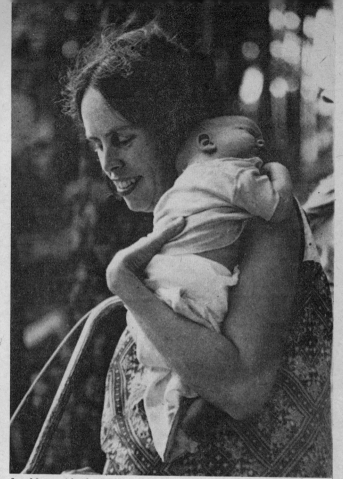

Ina May, midwife at The Farm, holding young Paul Benjamin. Many lay midwives today call themselves "empirical" midwives, trained by experience.

woman little more than reassurance, encouragement, guidance, and a pair of helping hands. We specialize in normal pregnancies and normal, spontaneous deliveries and provide total maternity care as part of a team practicing in hospitals or maternity homes with obstetricians who serve as emergency back-up in case of complications."

Kitty Ernst, CNM, of Maternity Center Association, New York, trained at the Frontier Nursing Service and also holds a degree in public health. She has contributed much to the establishment and

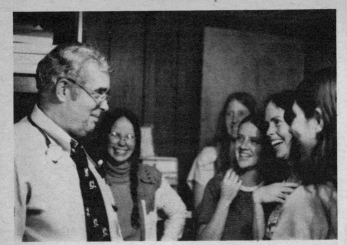

Midwives at The Farm meeting with Dr. John O. Williams, who provides medical backup and counsel. The midwives attend deliveries and run the Clinic at the Farm.

running of MCA's new Childbearing Center, in addition to her teaching and article-writing. In 1971, as a consultant from MCA, she helped to create Booth Maternity Center in Philadelphia, a single-class facility staffed by ten midwives and three obstetricians.

Midwives attend at deliveries at Booth and partake in other activities as well. Carol Paruch, of Nova Scotia, CNM from Meheary Hospital in Nashville, taught the prenatal class I attended at Booth this spring.

Another prominent educator—midwives are all educators, and most are also parents—is Ruth Wilf, CNM, who came to nurse-midwifery after preparation for her own labor in a CEA class. With her CNM colleagues at Booth, she is now on the planning team for the new home-birth facility there. She is also active with such organizations as the National Association of Parents & Professionals for Safe Alternatives in Childbirth (NAPSAC), and the Association of Childbirth at Home International (ACHI) (see Chapter 6).

Certified Nurse-Midwife Ruth Lubic, General Director of MCA, sees the importance of her profession ultimately in terms of the sense of trust which it strives to foster: "In my opinion, nurse-midwifery management of the entire childbearing experience offers an unusual opportunity for the establishment of trust between care receivers and care givers."

How does the presence of the CNM affect our obstetrical outcome, as clients? Nancy Mills, in the NAPSAC article previously quoted, reports the following:

"In Madero County, California, ten years ago [1966], the State supported a project that introduced midwives into that community. It was a very rural, low income community and lacked availability of any prenatal care. After one year, the infant mortality was reduced from 23.9 per 1000 live births to 10.3. Prematurity dropped from 11% of all births to 6.4%. These midwives obviously proved a great need for health care in that particular community. The project was dropped, at the recommendation of the Health Department and the obstetricians of the State. Within six months, the very high percentage of problems increased back to its normal of its unusually high rate that existed before the program was adopted."

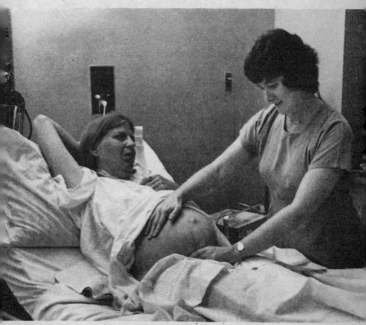

Barbara Brennan, Certified Nurse-Midwife at Roosevelt Hospital in New York, checks the position of a baby about to be born. Ms. Brennan was the first CNM to practice on a hospital staff in the United States—beginning in 1964.

Suzanne Arms (*Immaculate Deception*) gives us these two reports of results where the CNM is at work:

In Holmes County, Mississippi, the infant death rate decreased from 41.5 per 1000 live births to 21.3 per 1000, under nurse-midwife care over a three-year period.

A Maryland hospital study compared childbirth experiences of women having a nurse-midwife in attendance with outcomes for a similar group of women treated by a physician. The women treated by nurse-midwives had shorter labors; 90% gave birth without forceps. Among the doctor's patients, 58% had forceps deliveries.

To all concerned, reports roll in of the enthusiasm of parents for nurse-midwife services in hospitals and maternity centers. Women are traveling extra miles to find the kind of care they want; services in hospitals which have added nurse-midwives to their staff find that couples who could afford to go elsewhere are choosing to use the services which include nurse-midwifery.

Her ubiquity and the professional, organized manner of her practice are spurring a public consciousness of the nurse-midwife and an acceptance of midwifery in general. The result cannot but benefit all manner of midwives and their prospective clients.

DOCTORS AND THE OBSTETRICAL TEAM

Accepting a new concept of the obstetrical team by admitting to it this new professional, the CNM, is not easy. Obstetricians have grown used to a position of unchallenged primacy in their field, with nurses as their aides; and champions of independent midwifery tend to suspect the nurse-midwife of accepting a role as doctor's loyal assistant and no more. Taking the issue one step further, Suzanne Arms sees nursing and mid-wifery as incompatible in some respects. How, she asks, can the nurse-midwife, trained in the medical profession, be committed to the midwifely way of protecting the laboring woman from medical interference? Moreover, Arms criticizes the colleague relationship which the nurse-midwife develops with the physician, doubting that doctors will accept anyone but doctors into equal status with them.

Yet some doctors are glad for the change: "I like nurse-midwives and they make me comfortable so long as they don't begin to act like physicians," says pediatrician Robert Mendelsohn in *Safe Alternatives in Childbirth*.

Dr. Kloosterman, eminent Dutch obstetrician, says it this way: "In quite a number of situations, it is difficult to draw the line between normality and abnormality. In these situations, the obstetrician needs an experienced midwife who can act as his partner in the discussion and sometimes even as his conscience'' (reported by Arms).

During one visit with Dr. Franklin at Booth Maternity Center this spring, I asked about the benefits to obstetricians of the work of nurse-midwives.

The nurse-midwife, he said, gives assurance of labor support, something few doctors are trained for, interested in, or empowered by their schedule to do. A woman supported in labor is more relaxed and responsive—if obstetricians would exchange their preference for inert bodies to practice on for a new appreciation of the way a prepared and midwife-supported mother can help to insure a safe and successful outcome, the figures would be better. Incidentally, he added, what is felt to be a deception, a warping, in American birth, could straighten up and begin to show a positive trend in health care.

Many obstetricians are most skilled in that part of obstetrics which is technology-oriented, which sets about solving complications in labor and delivery. Their training, for centuries, has prepared them to expect to intervene, to perfect and extend those interventions. A talent in this area, however, does not noticeably correlate with sensitivity in the attending part of the obstetrical role, and why should it? It is hard to find individuals with skills in both areas.

Some obstetricians are primarily surgeons by temperament. Some are philosophers, crusaders, and theoreticians. Some are most of all like a GP, a general practitioner or family doctor. For some, the routine birth is boring; for others, it is the focus of their work. For some, the prospect of attending a home birth is their call (see Beatrice Tucker of Chicago Maternity Center, Chapter 5); and for others this prospect is horrifying. Some enjoy the presence of the father, some find him a nuisance.

Midwifery and obstetrics, the being-with and the standing-by, are not, after all, *rival* versions of one field of health care. They complement and/or supplement one another. It turns out that we need both approaches, plus a few, for in-depth maternity care.

In working out a good relationship with an obstetrician, you may wish to give some thought to why obstetricians and anesthesiologists tend to want to intervene in birth experience. *Our Bodies, Ourselves,* that excellent women's health book from Boston, suggests five general reasons to consider; I include them in slightly altered form:

(1) Doctors have their own notions about how painful labor is, and tend to see the experience as an ordeal from which women need to be rescued by doctors (this is even true of female doctors sometimes).

(2) Medical training teaches doctors to think in terms of complica-

tions; normal births are medically boring, complicated ones offer a challenge.

(3) In American medicine there is a notable worship of technology; doctors tend to feel that they are depriving their patients if they do not use the latest and the most sophisticated techniques and drugs.

(4) Doctors are acutely aware of the possibility of malpractice suits; that is, they want to use the most up-to-date techniques so that they can prove, if necessary, that they gave their "patient" the best possible care (in a sense, the insurance companies have something to do with the way labor is managed).

(5) Hospitals are understaffed and doctors are overworked: this tends to make personal attention for each woman difficult; there is, rather, a tendency to routinize procedures and to use monitoring machines instead of constant personal supervision.

In reassessing my own hospital birth-giving, I have been surprised at how many options were available to me, way back in 1969.

I went to visit with my obstetrician, and I asked him at the end of the visit how he had come to be so much involved with hypnosis and with techniques of natural childbirth at a time when most of his colleagues ignored or summarily resisted such practices. He just smiled, warm and weary. I saw that there isn't an answer to that, of course. It's just the way he is. He was the first doctor in his area to accept husbands in the labor and delivery rooms, and the first to use hypnosis. I was lucky to have happened upon an obstetrician whose personal approach included offering these kinds of options.

Obstetrical training is almost entirely medicine-oriented. How many medical students, even those specializing in ob/gyn, have witnessed unmedicated birth? Home birth? Even in films? Virtually none. Advance preparation and education on the part of the pregnant women are considered appropriate when combined with complete confidence in the obstetrical staff.

But the training of obstetricians is becoming, inevitably, subject to change. Midwives, indirectly, are participating in the broadening of obstetrical-care education: as midwives join the staffs of hospitals, medical students are influenced by their approach to various aspects of obstetrical care. Directly, nurse-midwives influence obstetrical training in their capacities as consultants and teachers in medical schools. Doctors who as residents worked with nurse-midwives are, Elliott McCleary reports in *New Miracles of Childbirth,* requesting nurse-midwifery collaboration in their new practices. (McCleary calls nurse-midwives "super-nurses.")

The obstetrical team, then, includes most noticeably the midwife and the obstetrician; but there are others.

Nurses who work on hospital maternity wards have sometimes had special training in obstetrics. Although their status relegates them to a secondary position in the field, such nurses often provide support to mothers, especially when nurse-midwives are absent. Nurses without special obstetrical training often also acquire midwifely skills, and give most welcome personal support to laboring women. The public-health nurse is the medical mainstay to large numbers of rural and urban dwellers.

In the delivery room, should a woman need or desire an anesthetic, it will most likely be administered by an anesthesiologist, a doctor with a specialty in anesthetic agents; within this specialty, obstetrical anesthesia is a subspecialty. This level of care is costly for hospitals and for individuals. The shortage of well-trained anesthesiologists is also a problem where anesthesia is a popular choice.

How does the pediatrician fit in with the idea of an obstetrical team?

In American medicine, the charge of the obstetrician is the health of the parturient woman. The baby, as long as it is a fetus, is also his responsibility. But as soon as the baby emerges, it becomes the concern of a different specialist, the pediatrician, sometimes a hospital-based pediatrician specializing in what is known as neonatology.

This separation of care-giving is convenient for the professionals, but not usually in the best interests of the care-receivers. Can we clearly separate into obstetric vs. pediatric responsibilities the infant emerging from the mother's body, the infant still connected by the cord as it lies nursing on its mother's belly, the newly separated infant, wriggling in the adjoining crib, who may or may not be requiring neonatal care while the mother is yet being watched for continuing contractions and the remainder of the afterbirth is being checked out? Clearly these are not easily separable concerns. They overlap. An integrated team approach to the event of parturition will at least give a much-needed continuity of care, and may in some cases prevent tragedy, as medical specialization may lead to a serious lack of communication among the various specialists.

Take, for example, this story. A young woman becomes pregnant. She is at the time being clinically treated for what has been diagnosed as depression. Her depression is chronic and severe enough to have warranted treatment with lithium, a strong drug used for relief of specific symptoms. Her obstetrician, of course, knows of this. She goes into labor, and in due time gives birth to an infant who at once shows striking symptoms of some disorder. The *pediatrician*, attributing the symptoms to one of several possible causes, begins to try to find an appropriate treatment. At the point of losing the baby, the pediatrician happens to ask the obstetrician if there is anything from his experience which would shed light on the crisis. The information about the lithium is crucial; the baby is saved, barely, from severe toxicity reactions.

Psychiatry, like pediatrics, is also a specialty which needs to be better integrated with obstetrical care.

This is not to say that all doctors should master several specialties, or even add materially to their already heavy workload. It is the issue of teamwork in the structure of the agency or institution where the doctors practice that is more relevant than any individual doctor's continuing training. Knowing when to refer an obstetrical patient to some particular medical or social-service resource is an art in itself, a practical art, sorely needed.

What midwifery offers is continuity of care for the mother, baby, and family as a unit. Should there be damage to the baby or conditions requiring immediate care, the presence of a medical specialist is, of course, essential and welcomed by the midwife.

Some other possible members of the obstetrical team may have titles which are found only in their particular hospital or facility—often these are experimental positions, attempted solutions to the problem of staffing. In the obstetrics ward of one of the two hospitals serving a small city in Ontario (Sault Ste.-Marie, population 80,000), there is a staff member known as a Mother's Nurse, whose role is to teach infant care. My friend who delivered at that hospital reports that this special nurse was a great help in "humanizing the staff-patient situation."

Vanderbilt University Hospital in Nashville, Tennessee, has on the staff an RN (Registered Nurse) whose title is Family Nurse Clinician. Her various responsibilities include interpreting, designing, and promoting the maternity program of the hospital, helping families adjust to the program, helping the program adjust to needs of particular clients, and helping to publicize the screening for high-risk/low-risk pregnancy; in the regionalization scheme, this high-risk center is known for its specialized work.

In the division of obstetrical labor, where does gender fit in? The issue, after all, is that of choosing, of selecting wherever possible a birth attendant who suits you. Obstetricians are males, 97% are; midwives in at least that high a percentage are female. In *The Experience of Childbirth*, Sheila Kitzinger, with her emphasis on the psychological aspects of childbearing, expresses the question of the gender of the birth attendant this way. Some women, she says, see the obstetrician as someone "who will be firm, authoritarian and kind, like a loving father. . . . Other women need their mothers with them. . . . The midwife may be a satisfactory mother substitute. . . . But, of course, not all women are like that. Many seek primarily a less highly charged relationship with the midwife—one in which the two can work as partners towards the safe and happy delivery of the baby. . . . a cooperative enterprise with a midwife whom they [mothers] look to as a specialist to inform them, quite openly and truthfully, of progress and delay, and to remind them of what they should be doing at each phase of labour.''

Of course, some women have grown comfortably with their long-standing relationship with a male doctor. One woman I know had for years been going to a particular obstetrician, a man, kindly—rather, I think, like Dr. Dick-Read himself, basically astonished by the miracle of it. One child, one divorce, and many Pap smears later, the woman joined a health plan which included gynecology, and she went with curiosity for a routine checkup with the female ob/gyn whom the health plan had newly on staff. Imagine the woman's surprise when the lady doctor, bright, cool, confident, and remote, checked her out as if she were some specimen, and the woman felt an immediate yearning for good old Dr. X, with his warmth and his relaxed ways.

Yet with the acceptance of midwives and the widening range of available maternity personnel, there is now more choice than ever for both the gender and genre of birthing attendants.

FATHERS

Very often, tribesmen participate in birth in the role of shaman or medicine man, appearing at times of emergency to enact important magical performances. Among the Dayak people of Borneo, recounts Milinaire in *Birth,* a magician and his assistant would visit a woman having a difficult labor. The assistant would stand outside the hut with a moon-colored stone tied to his belly; the magician, massaging and soothing the woman, would shout instructions to him to move the stone in imitation of the baby's movements, an act of magical substitution/transference.

Husbands, similarly, would participate in birth, enacting a kind of protective magic. The practice of *couvade,* explains Milinaire, is a serious decoy attempt to absorb or at least divide the interests of any malign powers: ''When the woman stops her daily activities to give birth, she will go either to a special birth house of the village or off into the countryside to give birth by herself and return a few hours later with babe in hand. The father, meanwhile, goes to his sleeping area and pretends to be greatly shaken and in need of attention, moaning and groaning. Sometimes the father will perform these ceremonial gestures for days before and after the actual birth.''

Today, in our society, it is becoming increasingly evident that men

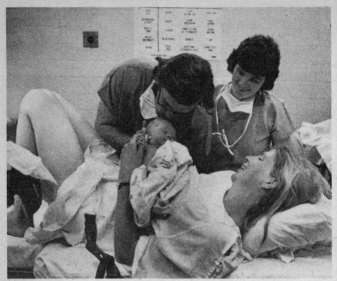

Father greets his very new child. A nurse-midwife attended at this hospital labor and delivery. Many hospitals allow fathers in the delivery rooms.

want to experience childbirth in their life, in the life of their woman companion or mate, in the life of the family they are creating. And women want them to. My friend and I, touring the hospital where sometime in the next week or two she would give birth, were delighted to see in every room a young father cradling his tiny offspring, identical looks of love and incredulity on their faces. Fathers are going to prenatal class, to prenatal check-ups, to labor, and to delivery. They are learning to offer a special, close support.

Feeling *with* the woman is at the heart of good midwifing. One may ask, how can the male truly empathize with the sensations of the laboring woman? Someone who has felt these sensations before can be more immediately intuitive, that's clear. But anybody can try. In the prenatal class I went to at Booth, the midwife, Carol, directed a role-reversal exercise. This gave the women a chance to show what kind of attending they would like, and gave the men a chance to put themselves in laboring shoes, just for a fantasy of a few minutes.

The man who supports his woman during labor is in a position in which the most he can know of her sensations is the best he can imagine them—but he has the reassurance of prenatal education to help him, and sometimes a labor guide sheet. He has the security, usually, of knowing that good medical backup is nearby, standing ready. And he has the exciting outcome of the event to buoy up his (and, thus, your) spirits. The more actively he can provide empathy, loving calm, and physical support, the more he will realize, later, the unique usefulness of his contribution to the success of the experience. The more that fathers embrace fathering, the nicer for everybody. Mothers need more help than they get, children need to know men in nurturing roles, and fathers deserve to experience active parenting of their infants, of which so many of them have been deprived.

During labor the father can mediate between his thoroughly concentrating wife and the often rapid, often unexplained medical whirl of the hospital labor and/or delivery rooms. He can translate her needs to the staff and arrange with the staff to proceed in a way that meets his woman's needs. He can bring to her the kind of confidence and loving support that can really help open up a scared cervix. In *Spiritual Midwifery* a laboring women expresses the feeling that the "love-making energy was what would open me up."

Of course, there are men who by temperament or cultural tradition do not want to participate in childbirth by being present during labor or at the delivery. Just as a woman who has planned labor unmedicated should be encouraged not to feel like a failure if she decides to ask for some relief, the prospective father who sits it out should be encouraged not to start his new paternity with a case of guilt.

Whether you will be allowed to bring your husband (or company of any kind) into the birthing place is of course determined by the institution. This is a matter you will want to work out with your attendant, and your institution, as pregnancy progresses. Smaller facilities adhere less rigidly to exclusion rules about such things. It is, however, becoming increasingly common in hospitals for fathers to be allowed to accompany wives in the labor room, and to a lesser extent in the delivery room as well. In some institutions it is a matter of policy that the husband leave when any heavy medication is to be administered to the laboring woman.

The surge of father-participation became noticeable with the appearance of Dr. Robert A. Bradley's *Husband-Coached Childbirth* in 1965. In this book Dr. Bradley, of Colorado, has developed and extended ideas of natural childbirth mostly from Dick-Read's work in presenting the case for the importance of the husband in the childbearing experience. *Husband-Coached Childbirth* is chatty and informal (sometimes perhaps overly so—I, for one, wince at hearing the uterus called the "baby box"), and, directed as it is toward men, makes a positive contribution toward the inclusion of the husband in the dynamics of pregnancy, labor, and postpartum adjustment.

Classes in Bradley's method stress the teaching of muscular relaxation while of course emphasizing the participation of the father as labor coach and main support. Dangers of drugs and interventions are also taught (there is a chapter in the revised edition called "It's Not Nice to Fool Mother Nature"). In 1965 Dr. Bradley had some encouraging statistics for his method: in 10,000 deliveries, 93.5% were unmedicated; no mothers or babies died. Bradley's publication was followed a few years later by the founding of the American Academy of Husband-Coached Childbirth (AAHCC) (see Chapter 6). The organization trains teachers in Bradley's method throughout the U.S.A. and elsewhere.

In 1938 Maternity Center Association began a series of classes for prospective fathers; there was a large response, and the syllabus was distributed from coast to coast. The next year MCA followed up with *Getting Ready to Be a Father*, a conversational and practical book.

Other books on the subject include Dr. George Schaefer's *The Expectant Father*, "a practical guide," less influenced by Dick-Read than *Husband-Coached Childbirth*, but not as satisfactory on the

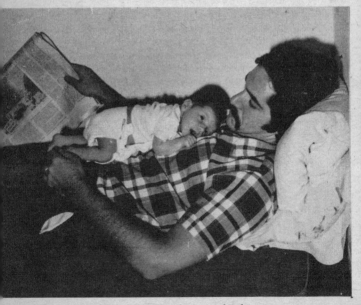

Father and daughter getting to know each other.

emotional issues as Bradley. Peter Mayle, author of the excellent children's books *Where Did I Come From?* (about conception) and *What's Happening To Me?* (about puberty), has just issued a new book called *How To Be a Pregnant Father*. In the collaborative work *Pregnancy, The Psychological Experience,* Arthur and Libby Colman discuss the stages of pregnancy, and labor and delivery in the context of the experience of the expectant father as well as the expectant mother. One section, entitled "Emotional Problems of the Expectant Father," discusses "running away" as "the most common behavioral problem."

THE ART OF THE MIDWIFE

Midwifery is as ancient as birth-giving. Much of what the modern midwife does is what midwives always have done. To sum up, we will enumerate the universal features of her work.

(1) *She keeps company.*

From one of the earliest texts, *The Byrthe of Mankynde* (1540): "Also the midwife must struct and comfort the partie, not onely refreshing her with good meate and drinke, but also with sweete woordes, gevying her good hope of a speedfull deliverance."

There has never been a culture that left women alone or with strangers during labor—except for ours between about 1930 and about 1960, the heyday of standard American hospital birth. The midwife's very name tells us she will stay with us. The comfort of this knowledge can affect our labor: While showing a film of a sympathetic midwife managing at a hospital birthing, the eminent Dutch obstetrician Dr. Naaktgeboren commented that "the telepathic effect of a good word can be as powerful as oxytocin" (quoted by Arms).

Keeping company need not be limited to verbal activity. A belly dancer from Buffalo, New York, suggests that belly dancing had its origins in an ancient matriarchal fertility ritual. The dance's sensuous "belly rolls" are imitations of uterine contractions, practice for childbirth, sympathetic magic, suggests Daniela Gioseffi ("Lifting the Veil of Isis," *Quest*). Tribeswomen in the Middle East, even in this century, would dance around the laboring woman to hypnotize her into relaxing with contractions.

(2) *She studies to learn more, and she teaches.*

Louise Bourgeois, "the first great woman practitioner of obstetrics," as Adrienne Rich calls her, trained midwives and taught obstetrics to surgeons. From her text of 1609 comes this model charge: "Undertake, till the last day of life, to learn; which to do readily requires a great humbleness, for the proud do not win the hearts of those who know secrets. Never in your life venture to employ any medicine in which you have been instructed, neither on the poor nor on the rich, unless you are certain of its virtue and that it can do no harm, whether taken within the body or applied upon it'' (quoted by Rich).

The Farm says it this way: "A midwife must be an avid student of physiology and medicine. You should read and study constantly in a never-ending quest for new information."

Ruth Lubic, CNM: "Education of mothers and families is the soul of nurse-midwifery practice."

(3) *She feels a personal responsibility, a calling.*

From the Farm: "The midwife's job is to do her best to bring both the mother and child through their passage alive and stoned and to see that the sacrament of birth is kept Holy. (Stoned is defined as "charged with spiritual energy" by the authors of *Spiritual Midwifery*.) The Vow of the Midwife has to be that she will put out one hundred per cent of her energy to the mother and the child that she is delivering until she is certain that they have safely made the passage. This means that she must put the welfare of the mother and child first, before that of herself and her own family, if it comes to a place where she has to make a choice of that kind" (*Spiritual Midwifery*).

Guatemalan midwife Etta Willis spoke at the El Paso conference about the work of the midwife: "I always put this in my midwife's head: that she is an important person in her community. The thing of being an important person is not that it gives her the right to be higher than the people. She has to share love first, and after she has to share compassion for the people. Don't hide what you have in your heart, because not everyone was born to be a midwife. A midwife is something special, it's given to us from God. It's born into you to be a midwife. You feel it to be a midwife. Only God gives us that, and He doesn't charge us anything. He gives it up to us free. Let's be sisters, let's be brothers and work together to help the people."

(4) *She does not charge high fees.*

Louise Bourgeois, midwife and teacher, wrote in 1609 that the midwife should collect as small a fee as possible from the poor, "for little may seem much to them."

Lay midwife Nancy Mills: "I don't have a specific midwifery fee. Very often families ask me how much I charge. I usually say, 'It's whatever you can afford.' . . . The personal rewards are what keeps me going."

The Farm midwives say: "We practice free spiritual midwifery

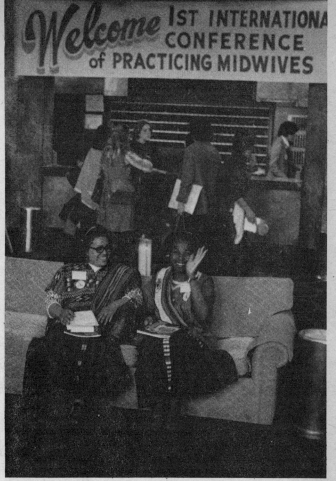

Guatemalan midwives Blanca de Colindres and Etta Willis at the El Paso Conference for practicing midwives in early 1977.

because it gives us a clean moral position if we need to talk to a lady about her attitude or tell her to stop complaining.''

Mrs. Andy Webb, granny-midwife: ''I'd rather have a midwife anytime as a doctor. They know their business, and a doctor don't care. . . . He might do somethin' to help your back, and then he'll reach out and get your pocketbook and that's all he wants. When I get in pain and get t'hurtin' or get sick, th'midwife's th'one to go to.

That's th'only one will help anybody if they ain't got a big pocketbook'' (*Foxfire 2*).

To this listing of venerable traits we should add that the modern midwife, while practicing with medical backup, continues to respect and protect childbirth as a natural process.

Suzanne Arms: ''The midwife begat the obstetrician, as it was the midwife who practiced for thousands of years in a world where birth was regarded as a natural and normal function of the human body.''

From the first issue of *The Practicing Midwife*, a newsletter emerging from the El Paso conference, attended by doctors, midwives, nurse-midwives, nurses, writers, and parents: ''The conference discussed ideas like the role of the midwife as a protector of normal birth; the need for developing good midwife-hospital relations (especially for handling an occasional emergency); the delicate bonding procedure which occurs between mother and child; and the way a midwife can manage the energy released in childbirth so as to have a successful, uncomplicated, fulfilling experience for everyone involved.''

* * *

SOME MILESTONES IN THE DEVELOPMENT OF MODERN MIDWIFERY

1918 Maternity Center Association opens in New York

1922 First class for fathers at MCA

1925 Midwife Mary Breckinridge opens the Frontier Nursing Service in Kentucky

1932 First school for nurse-midwives, the Lobenstine Clinic, established in New York

1939 Sculptures of stages of labor on view at World's Fair in New York attract thousands; these are pictured in Maternity Center Association's *Birth Atlas*

1945 Midwives licensed for the first time, in New Mexico

1947 Grantly Dick-Read speaks in this country under the auspices of MCA

1950 First reports on Natural Childbirth, from a study by Yale University and MCA, show that labor is more comfortable, shorter, less tiring, and accompanied by less bleeding when natural childbirth methods are used

1955 American College of Nurse-Midwifery (ACNM) established

1964 Nurse-midwives begin practicing in hospitals (Roosevelt Hospital in New York)

1971 Booth Maternity Center established in Philadelphia; Santa Cruz Birth Center established in California

1974 There are over 100 nurse-midwifery services in the country; ACNM moves to Washington, D.C.; midwives are arrested at Santa Cruz for practicing medicine without a license

1975 MCA opens its Childbearing Center

1977 January, First International Conference of Practicing Midwives, El Paso, Texas

1978 Over 20 nurse-midwifery services in New York City alone

1979 "The Five Standards for Safe Childbearing"—A NAPSAC Conference in Nashville and on The Farm

5

Birth Place

In the United States and Canada the vast majority of births take place in hospitals. Estimates I have heard are in the 90-to-95 percent range. This is a recent development, historically.

The home was and is the primary birth place among primitive people. (The second most common place for tribal folk was the birthing hut, a special place designated for birth alone, or shared with menstruating women.) With institutionalization in the European Middle Ages came the development of Lying-In hospitals, the first hospital-like facilities for maternity care. The Lying-In hospital was not an institution for the sick and injured.

At the turn of the twentieth century in the United States, a majority of individuals still gave birth at home. In 1915 in Manhattan a study analyzing obstetrical care estimated that 35% of women delivered in a hospital. The percentage from rural areas would, of course, have been much lower. Worldwide, 98% of the people *alive today*, report Marion Sousa (*Childbirth at Home*) and others, were born at home. As the science of obstetrics grew, and independent midwifery declined in favor, hospital birth became the North American way. And so it has remained for some decades.

Yet as ideas about natural childbirth have spread, as the practice of standardized obstetrical management has been scrutinized, and as modern-day midwifery services have become more widespread, many people have felt a desire or need to experience childbirth apart from the structures of hospital routine. In the United States, the movement toward home birth has been growing in popularity—the old way has become a "new" option. In addition, the idea of the maternity center is now blooming as another increasingly available option. Variety is becoming the rule of the day; as consumers of childbirth care, we all stand to benefit from this trend.

This chapter looks at choices for facilities in which to give birth— the hospital, the home, and the maternity center. Necessarily, there is some degree of overlap in the presentation of ideas relevant to each choice such that the information and the personal accounts should be digested as a unit of thought before making any final assessments about choice of birth place. What is most important to emphasize is that in selecting a birth place we are choosing more than just a room; we are choosing a kind of maternity care, placing ourselves in a more-or-less predictable continuum of control. The stories recounted here of birth at home and birth at a maternity center fit most descriptions of how birthings in those settings generally occur; there are no startling discrepancies. The hospital birth story, though, is strikingly uncharacteristic of what descriptions of hospital birth would lead us to expect. From this we can take heart, I believe: there are ways *not* to be deceived, immaculately or otherwise, even if we choose a hospital for our labor and delivery.

HOSPITAL BIRTH

Giving birth in a hospital, we have noted, is a relatively new idea. Once it caught on in this country during the second quarter of the century, it spread and grew and knew no competition. Vogue played a part in the way women made such choices, as indeed it was plainly more fashionable to go to the hospital to give birth. Along with this trend it was also more in fashion for babies to be bottle-fed—home birth and breastfeeding were regarded as lowerclass choices by the great hospital-going majority.

General features: benefits and risks

The one overwhelming benefit of giving birth in a hospital is the security of medical help in the event of trouble. This is a medical benefit, therefore, and it is also for many a psychological benefit.

Management of labor in which there is any complication, such as those described in Chapter 3, is best conducted in a well-equipped hospital obstetric unit. Complication arises in approximately 1 out 10 labors.

The risks of this choice of birth place take more telling.

American hospital birth has been described many times over, often in anger and in criticism. Doris Haire's *The Cultural Warping of Childbirth* and Suzanne Arms' *Immaculate Deception*—their attitudes are explicit in the titles—are important, pioneering works that give us a basis for vigilance. At the heart of Arms' study is what she sarcastically refers to as the "The New, Improved, Quick-and-Easy, All-American Hospital Birth." According to Richard and Dorothy Wertz, authors of the soon-to-be published *Lying-In: A History of*

Childbirth in America, much of the safety and joy of the social and wholesome tradition of home birthing has been lost over the generations to standardized and impersonal hospital routines.

When you enter a hospital, you should understand that you are accepting a medical environment and a medical orientation toward childbirth. This means that there is a much greater overall likelihood that medicine will be practiced on you even if your labor progresses normally without any medical problems whatever. Hospitals exist for treatment of sickness. This is reassuring for those who are concerned with complications and for those who must favor the medical environment. For others, who see birth primarily as a natural bodily process and a family event, these medical surroundings may be a cause for dismay.

Doris Haire, past president of the International Childbirth Education Association, lists and describes the standard features which led her to regard American hospital birth as a warping. It is these factors individually and especially in combination which may be called the "risks" of hospital birth, although obviously not all the factors always pertain to any given hospital. Here is Haire's list, adapted.

1. Attitudes: information regarding disadvantages of medications and procedures is not usually offered; mothers are not encouraged to help themselves work with their labors.

2. Elective induction of labor; routine stimulation of labor by oxytocics.

3. Confinement of the laboring woman to bed; moving of mother from labor bed to delivery room; requiring the flat-on-back, strapped-down position for delivery.

4. Overenthusiastic use of medication and technology where it is not medically required.

5. Routine shaving of pubic area; routine use of forceps; routine episiotomy; routine early clamping of umbilical cord; routine suctioning of the newborn's air passages.

6. Obstetrical intervention in expulsion of placenta.

7. Interference with and nonsupport of breastfeeding.

8. Prevention of early father-child contact; restriction of rooming-in.

9. Routine separation of mother from newborn, each to separate recovery facility and separate medical supervision; also, separation of mother from family.

This last item, perhaps in the long run the most serious aspect of warping in American childbirth, warrants some elaboration here. Indeed, separation was the watchword in the heyday of routine hospital birth—and it still is where those practices remain unchallenged. In this model, to give birth a woman must separate from her partner, the father of the baby, and from all of her family. She is separated from her own consciousness and sense of control by a battery of routine medication and procedures administered usually without explanation. Then she is separated from her baby immediately after birth, preventing the experience of immediate acquaintance with the baby. We are aware that maternal feelings grow gradually, and that even severe separation is not necessarily followed by permanent impairment of the mother-child relationship. Still, once the nature of bonding after birth is understood at all, it is hard to imagine holding on to policies which actively discourage this. The entire separation phenomenon is the topic of Klaus and Kennell's study *Maternal-Infant Bonding,* and is an issue of grave concern for Dr. Leboyer in *Birth Without Violence.*

The disadvantages associated with most of the routines listed above have been discussed in the preceding chapters. Birthing position (item 3), a factor over which hospitals exert considerable control, we have not yet examined.

In early first-stage labor, most women are most comfortable moving around. As contractions become stronger and require more concentration, a sitting or semi-sitting position is usually the most appropriate choice. Yet many hospitals still expect women to take all of labor and delivery lying down.

The supine position—flat on the back, feet usually up in stirrups—is known technically as the *lithotomy* position. Introduced in the 17th century when the new vogue for male doctor birth attendants appeared, this position offers the attendant a good view. A standard, contemporary obstetrical textbook still presents it this way: under the heading "Position For Delivery," the sub-heading is "Lithotomy Position" and the entry reads, "The lithotomy position is the best. . . . The patient is in the ideal position for the attendant to deal with any complications which may arise" (Oxorn and Foote, *Human Labor and Birth,* 1975).

Dr. Roberto Caldeyro-Barcia (president of the International Federation of Gynecologists and Obstetricians, the director of the Latin American Center for Perinatology and Human Development of the World Health Organization) disagrees unequivocally: "Except for being hanged by the feet," he states, "the supine position is the worst conceivable position for labor and delivery."

Doris Haire reports some reasons why the supine position is medically a problem. She points out that this position tends to: (1) adversely affect the mother's blood pressure by compressing the vena cava, thus reducing the rate of blood flow to the fetus; (2) decrease intensity of contractions; (3) inhibit the mother's natural, voluntary effort to push the baby out, thus increasing the need for forceps and

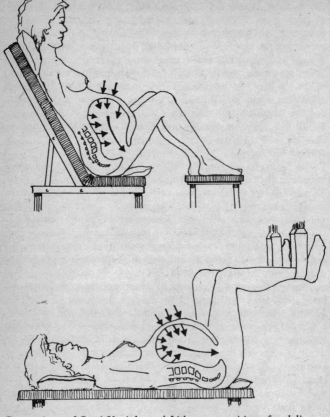

Comparison of Semi-Upright and Lithotomy positions for delivery, with arrows indicating the force of gravity in each case.

increasing the amount of traction necessary for forceps extraction; (4) inhibit spontaneous expulsion of the placenta and thus increase the incidence of hemorrhage because of the need for pulling on the cord and/or manually extracting the placenta; and (5) increase the need for episiotomy because of tension on the pelvic floor.

Furthermore, it is obvious that gravity works *with* the efforts of the woman who is sitting or propped, works against the laboring of the woman flat on her back.

The supine position for delivery is rarely adopted by women who are choosing for themselves, as in home delivery, and according to accounts from other cultures. Midwives in Western Europe traditionally brought obstetrical stools with them: these were small chairs lacking most of the seat part so that the laboring woman could be mostly upright, supported, and the baby could be easily caught. Another person's lap was used similarly, sometimes the parturient's husband's. Until the 19th century, some degree of sitting up was the standard birthing position.

Pre-modern texts stress respect for and convenience of the woman. From *The Byrthe of Mankynde*, 1540, by Thomas Raynalde, a translation of sorts from a still earlier work: "The thynges which helpe the byrth and make it more easie, are these. First the woman that laboureth must eyther sytte groveling or els upright, leaning backwards, according as it shall seeme commodius and necessary to the partie, or as she is accustomed. . . ."

And, three centuries later, from the *Midwife's Practical Directory*, published in 1836 in Baltimore: "In giving manual assistance to a woman in labor, her own choice and convenience may commonly be consulted, in relation to the position in which she shall be placed. If any arrangement appears necessary, contrary to her inclinations, such arrangement should be suggested and made with tenderness and caution. The mild art of persuasion will often succeed, where the imperious assumption of authority, and a spirit of coercion, would meet with an unconquerable repulse."

Home birth pictures and accounts show that the kneeling and all-fours positions are often the choice of the mother. Squatting, which requires a considerable amount of strength, is another frequent choice. Elisabeth Bing estimates that two-thirds of the world's women still give birth squatting.

In hospitals and maternity centers where policy permits, most mothers are most comfortable in late first-stage and all of second-stage labor in a half-sitting position, propped by pillows. If the baby is coming too quickly, lying on the side is useful to lessen the force of gravity, making it easier to hold back on pushing in this position.

Labor-delivery beds with adjustable backs, the European style, are beginning to appear here. Manchester Memorial Hospital in Manchester, Connecticut, has introduced such beds in the special "Lamaze Rooms"; Caesarean rates are estimated to be half that of births in the traditional part of the hospital.

The prevalence of the lithotomy position, then, when compared with the alternatives, provides a sound example of what Doris Haire means by the warping of childbirth.

Fortunately, however, not all of the standardized features listed by

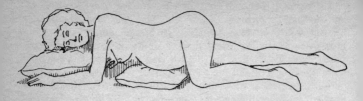

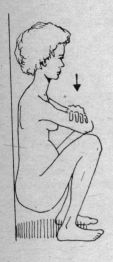

Alternative positions for labor. The side-lying position is usually more comfortable than the supine. Squatting for delivery utilizes gravity, though it usually requires a support for the woman to hold on to. A third alternative is the hands and knees position shown on page 44.

Haire as contributing to the "risks" of hospital birth are always present in each hospital setting. Nor are they all always risks; sometimes (see Chapter 3) an episiotomy is a relief. But together, as practiced *routinely*, they add up to an inauspicious portrait of childbirth in a great many North American hospitals.

We need to remember that not everyone is ready to abandon hospital birth. And it would not be wise to suggest that everyone should. Some of us are not comfortable about safety out-of-hospital; for large numbers of childbearing adults, it is unlikely that an ingrained belief in the ultimate security of hospitals will be dislodged. For many individuals the psychological comfort of giving birth in a hospital will ease anxieties which might otherwise be present and thus allow the laboring woman as worry-free an experience as possible. And, of course, even though the hospital birth rate has declined somewhat in the mid-seventies, the hospital is bound to continue managing the majority of births until alternative facilities and services become equally abundant. Furthermore, the American hospital, especially its out-patient clinic, is the "choice" for many couples who, unless they desire home birth, do not have the economic freedom to select at all.

For those of us who will, for whatever reasons, be going to the hospital when labor establishes itself, it is important to know how to make the most out of the childbearing experience there. For the point is not to itemize the "risks" and then panic, but simply to recognize these factors and exert your own educated preferences in order to insure that you get what you want in your childbirth. There is a variety in the hospital experience, and for everyone—including the poor, who are traditionally given the fewest options—there are ways to persist, to have a voice, to make changes, to be treated as a person and not just another case. It is no surprise that childbirth education classes often spend considerable class time discussing how to deal with hospitals. This can be an art in itself. Here are some clues and pieces of advice.

As so many commentators have recommended, the time to make your arrangements, the time to make known your own particular needs, the time to establish that you do not wish to be subject to routines or automatic standing orders is during pregnancy, from the start and regularly throughout. Flat on your back in the labor bed, coping on the edge of your control with the titanic contractions of transition, is no time to attempt a negotiation about routine I.V.

Many a busy obstetrician makes use of *standing orders,* that is, procedures and medications which he favors and uses routinely, which a nurse will administer in his absence. It is your right to know what your doctor's standing orders are. Early in your relationship with your doctor you should, if you wish, communicate the idea that your labor and delivery not be subject to standing orders, but managed according to its actual features.

What you need for hospital birth is what you need for any other place of birth: labor support, constancy of companionship. No society except ours in this century has ever sustained a tradition of leaving laboring women alone. Now this trend seems to have ended, as all obstetrical practice has at last come to appreciate how much more of a burden it is for the laboring person to be alone, how constant support is the simplest and most basic of pain-control measures. Luckily, this is one request that most hospitals honor. Fathers are so far making it to labor and delivery in hospitals. If you want someone other than the father to be with you, a firm but patient request has a chance of being granted. As the issue of being accompanied seems to be resolved, you will be simply stretching a detail.

Given all we know of medications, and all the evidence of greater safety and satisfaction when they are kept to a minimum, be forewarned that there are still many hospitals where pain-killing agents and/or oxytocics are given to laboring women without their consent. This is part of the view which sees checking in at the hospital as checking your control at the door. This means that some women, unsuspecting, suddenly find a gas mask held over their nose and mouth as the baby is crowning, or later learn that the I.V. drip which they though contained glucose had been used to administer Pitocin. Some doctors have a hard time relinquishing such procedures; your prenatal insistence, emphatic but calm, can remove the possiblity that you will have such a generally upsetting experience. Again, this is not to say that a whiff of gas for discomfort is a pernicious choice: it is the *unannounced* administration of any drug or procedure that you will probably wish to avoid.

Be aware that there could be a problem of inconsistency between your doctor's policies and the hospital's policies. Just because your doctor is enthusiastic about breastfeeding, or rooming-in, or your being allowed to walk around during early labor, it does not necessarily follow that the hospital encourages or even permits such practices. It will be up to you to follow through on these issues for your own protection. There is much potential confusion for a parent who gets a sense from childbirth education class of what is possible, likely, or unavoidable, and then finds once labor is underway that the doctor, despite his or her verbal support of the parents' wishes during pregnancy, is unable or unwilling to intercede to change hospital policy. Choice of hospital and choice of birth attendant are thus often intertwined. If the hospital where your doctor is on staff is inflexible, unwilling to respect your wishes, rather than fight your way through pregnancy it would be more productive to give them both up and find a new doctor-hospital arrangement that is responsive to your preferences.

To arrange your hospital birth to include the kind of management you want, *try to get your wishes and concerns noted on your chart*. This is standard policy at a family-centered facility like Booth Maternity Center, where your chart is a cumulative record of your health, the medicine you have been using, and your feelings and wishes as they develop during the period of pregnancy. In a standardized hospital, especially in a clinic situation where you do not see the same doctor each visit and cannot predict who will be the attendant at your birth, this effort to make your chart as precise as possible is particularly important. Wanting your wishes noted on the chart is NOT an attempt to take over the doctor's role or to be interfering. It would be a mistake to let yourself be talked into this version of your legitimate concern.

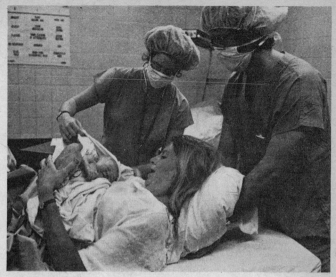

Hospital birth, immediately postpartum. Father-assisted, nurse-midwife attended.

Perhaps the single most important issue to pre-arrange with your hospital is that of staying together with your baby once he or she is born. Your ability as a mother, as parents, to accept and nurture this new dependent person in your life is clearly enhanced by getting to know one another in the same physical, attachment-fostering way that animals do (as the work of Klaus and Kennell describes). If you and your child are separated unnecessarily for the first 24 hours after birth, as is far from unusual in most hospital routines, you are being deprived of the best close and warm start for your new relationship. Being close with your baby during the time you are in the hospital means you can begin at once, when the infant's need for physical reassurance is all-important, to get used to handling him or her, often under the helpful supervision of the hospital staff. Rooming-in has been growing as a hospital option open to a variety of schedules, complete and partial. From the start of pregnancy, be specific about this issue with your obstetrician, be specific with the hospital pediatrician, who may well be the person who could alter a set policy, and be specific, too, with the maternity ward staff at the hospital wherever you can. This will help you get the schedule you want.

Don't hesitate to ask about hospital policy regarding *all* issues that are imporant to you. Use a checklist for your concerns, as is recommended also in selecting an obstetrician.

● *Talk to lots of people, evaluate their experiences.*

● *Read books.*

● *See yourself as a consumer.*

● *Express your preferences clearly to prospective attendants.*

Variations; regionalization

We have been describing hospital birth as if it were a monolithic, single-standard business. Actually, of course, there is a spectrum of size and orientation among hospitals. Further, some hospitals are now introducing within their walls variations in birth-place choice that resemble home-style, family-oriented, maternity centers (see beginning of Maternity Center section of this chapter for a representative description). And, significantly, within hospitals there are class diferences between clinic patients (usually poor) and private patients (usually less poor).

Generally speaking, these two observations hold up:

(1) The larger the hospital and the more closely affiliated with medical student education, the higher are its rates of maternal and infant mortality (see Haire on this).

(2) The larger and especially the more crowded the facility, the less likely it is that you will be able to secure deviations from routine procedures; you will have to be particularly persistent.

Clinic birth usually means less individual attention and no one attendant as a constant; rather, there is random assignment to obstetrical residents and the usually shifting nursing staff.

Some hospitals, such as the one where I had my daughter 8 years ago, are attempting to close the gap between clinic patients and private patients. My obstetrician now reports that clinic patients are receiving much more prenatal instruction than previously and are having the company of their husbands in labor and delivery. The overall effect is still, however, that of two classes of care.

Shaun's mother is expecting her second child any day now, her second and last, she says. She has chosen an Osteopathic Hospital with its small maternity unit for his birth, and has found it, so far, to be considerate and helpful. When I asked her about Shaun's birth, she winced and described how as a DPA (Department of Public Assistance) patient she had felt as if the clinic (at a large urban teaching hospital) had treated her like a cow. "I'm a college graduate, I've helped run a health clinic!'' and she gestured in frustration. ''They act as if you understand nothing if you are a DPA patient.'' She is allergic to most of the kinds of anesthetic and analgesic agents available to the laboring woman: over her protest they had injected a tranquilizer immediately upon her entering the hospital, assuming, evidently, that she could not be accurate about her own allergies.

This is not just a single, isolated incident of prejudiced behavior. It is a well documented fact that the poor are subjected to experimental procedures and medications often without their knowledge. An up-to-date, carefully researched study of women as medical guinea pigs is presented in Barbara Seaman's new book, *Women and the Crisis in Sex Hormones*.

In the occasionally topsy-turvy world of maternity care, on the other hand, there are sometimes unexpected benefits to birth at less well-endowed facilities. Two examples:

Nurse-midwifery came first to the out-patient clinic of Roosevelt Hospital in New York in 1964; now women well able to afford private care are choosing this service because they like nurse-midwifery attendance.

Many hospital outcomes document that obstetric patients at clinic have at times been given fewer routine drugs than their better-heeled sisters in private care, and in those cases fewer of their infants had drug-induced distress at birth.

A major effort in the political/geographical reorganization of maternity care resources is currently underway in the U.S. and Canada. This development, *regionalization*, aims to concentrate equipment and resources for high-risk obstetrics in one center per region while designating other facilities as either middle-level or small. Regionalization has implications for our choices as consumers.

The outline for this regionalization effort is presented in a pamphlet entitled ''Toward Improving the Outcome of Pregnancy'' prepared by a group called Committee on Perinatal Health. The working committee included no midwives, no nurse-midwives, no female doctors— only male M.D.s. (Six of the eight consultants on Personnel issues are women, one of them a CNM.)

The suggestions of the committee present a resource allocation whereby the high-risk centers would receive concentrated attention and funding. Maintenance of smaller facilities, low-risk-oriented hospitals, would receive little support or notice, except from consumers, of course, and from that portion of the obstetrical establishment which has such issues at heart (perhaps 10% at most).

Doris Haire describes regionalization this way in the 1976 NAPSAC report: ''Most of the world's women give birth at home or in a small maternity home attended by a midwife; yet there is a drive in the U.S. to eliminate small obstetric units and consolidate American obstetric services in order to justify the high cost of expensively equipped and staffed intensive care units.'' She further remarks that this is another example of ''the American penchant for adapting the entire system to meet the needs of the exceptions rather than the needs of the majority.''

The obstetric units of small community hospitals stand to lose much as a result of the regionalization drive. That would mean a great loss to many individuals, as small community hospitals are now among the more pleasant and responsive medical places at which to give birth. The story of Loretta and Zak is a model of well-planned, community-hospital birth. Compare it with the ''cut-yank-sew,'' rushed, routinized, medicated stories you can read in *Immaculate Deception*. The comparison will indicate the spectrum.

Story: Loretta and Zak

Chestnut Hill Hospital is a small, non-teaching facility designed to serve its own community. Late in March, I went with Loretta to the Hospital Tour class of the prenatal preparation series, the class where they explain how to navigate the actual arrival and stay at the hospital.

At this hospital, husbands are welcome. With some easy arranging, I was to be welcome, too.

Prepping there includes taking of blood pressure, pulse, and respiration, doing a fetal heart check, timing of contractions, and doing an internal exam for dilation. Pubic shave can be complete or ''mini'' (that is, a clipping instead of a shaving)—the woman must request her preference.

At Chestnut Hill Hospital there are three labor rooms, two doubles and a single; they are reasonably large. The beds are standard and the walls, colored in the omnipresent institutional green, are decorated here and there with little hanging objects and pictures which parents have left as focus items. The hospital has one fetal heart monitor per two labor beds; these are not used ''routinely.''

During labor there are regular checks and timings of progress. In the labor rooms there is a bell for calling the nurse (but this facility is so small that you could just raise your voice a little and the nurse would hear you). Women are hooked up to I.V. in the event that they turn out to need an anesthetic. During labor, women are encouraged to move around.

Delivery takes place in the delivery room, on a table with an adjustable back and a portion that slides to make a short, extended table for the birth itself. You stay on the delivery table for an hour or so, husband with you, while your blood pressure is checked, and the settling down of the uterus is watched. At this hospital Pitocin or Ergotrate is used to encourage postpartum contractions. Then, back in your room, you are bathed (this will feel wonderful, the teacher said) and may eat. The rooms are semi-private. At Chestnut Hill Hospital you are expected to stay for five days (standard), with the usual rounds of baby being brought in, checks by medical staff, visitors (evening visiting is restricted to fathers only). Rooming-in is available from 9 A.M. until 9 P.M.

Rooming-in procedures are much less rigid than before. You can have 24-hour rooming-in if you want it, said the orientation woman, but, she added, most mothers are glad to have a chance to get some sleep. Rooming-in babies have their own nursery, and parents may choose their level of involvement in infant care during the first few days. Please, the woman emphasized to expectant fathers, please wash hands carefully before handling your new baby—it took so long to get permission for fathers to participate, we don't want to throw any monkey wrenches in! A sickness can really spread in a nursery; don't handle the baby if you have any condition at all that might be catching.

This hospital sees 800 to 900 babies born a year, a large number for a community hospital.

I asked the young obstetric nurse at the desk if most parents get preparation classes. Yes, lots do, she answered. And, I asked, is there a difference in their experiences, do you think, as a result? A hundred-percent different, she declared; being prepared, having some idea of what will be happening, makes ALL the difference.

Prenatal classes at this hospital begin every six weeks. They are described as Lamaze style, a modified general breathing and exercise routine, plus general CEA-type physiological information. They are not taught by a certified Lamaze instructor.

Loretta and Zak had been taking a privately-run, standard Lamaze class. It was purposeful and serious, they say, which they found reassuring. They practiced conscientiously twice every day, breathing for the various stages of labor, relaxing certain parts of the body and tensing others. Their teacher, Marie Larello, well known in her field, has been educating couples for 15 years. Her pamphlet, which Loretta and Zak brought to the labor room, is called (after Dr. Lamaze's book) "Childbirth Without Pain." It is a clear summary of the exercises, breathing patterns, and postpartum exercise suggestions. Part of Larello's teaching emphasizes now to deal firmly with hospitals in planning for childbirth. (Marie Larello has also made a series of phonograph records with the basic Lamaze instructions—enormously helpful, I would imagine, for parents geographically unable to get to classes).

That was the preparation.

April 12, 1977, the first in what would be a string of days of perfect weather, clear and bright. Zak called me at 8:20 that morning. Loretta was in labor.

I arrived at Loretta and Zak's house near the river around 9:30. The three of us have been dear friends for years. For five hours we visited, drank cool white wine, played throw-the-stick with the dog (who never tires of it), and walked along the river by the house. We rolled up our sleeves and cuffs and drank in the April sunshine.

Loretta was having occasional mild contractions, and regular diarrhea, which was unpleasant.

The only time I saw Loretta off-balance during early labor was when another friend stopped by, then a couple of neighbor children, and then another neighbor lady with her dog. Loretta found all this activity too much—her concentration had been interrupted. Disoriented from her task, somewhat bewildered, she fled, in tears, into the house. For the body's work during early labor is under delicate control. Though the real drama of labor is yet to come, this early, preparatory stage requires concentration, effort, and privacy just to stay relaxed. Once you are relaxed, you tune in to the body's messages. My friend's inner sensors had told her that these unexpected stimuli were all too disruptive.

By 2:30, Loretta was having contractions, with back pain, at 6 or 7 minutes apart: On the phone, Dr. Kurtz suggested she come to the hospital. Bloody show and diarrhea had continued since morning. Loretta was breathing slow and deep and relaxing during contractions (which were lasting maybe 45 seconds). She preferred to be quiet, and lightly massaged her belly in a slow rhythmical way (effleurage). The back pain was her only real discomfort during this time.

We closed the suitcase, collected the bag of Lamaze stuff (like lollipops and talcum powder), said goodbye to the dog, and climbed into the van.

Loretta was not pleased to be jiggled around in the car. During contractions and between them the whole abdomen is very tender, and she wished Zak would go slow and not take bumpy roads.

At the Maternity Floor we met Dr. Kurtz and separated—Loretta to be checked and mini-prepped, Zak and I to wait in the little lounge.

After chatting in the lounge with a two-day mother, who spoke well of the care she had received at this hospital, we walked back to the labor room where Loretta—beautiful as always, in a light cotton hospital gown adorned with little blue flowers—had been installed. This labor room contained only the one bed; also a sink, a couple of chairs, a private bathroom, a window looking out over the city from what turns out to be the Hill part of Chestnut Hill.

All was peaceful. A young nurse came in friendly and quiet. We settled down and then talked. The nurse helped arrange pillows behind Loretta's back. We all sipped ice water.

From then, 3:00 or so, until we rolled on down the hall to the delivery room around 7:45, passed the final parts of the first stage of labor. During this time the nurse came in occasionally, listened to the heartbeat of the baby with her manual stethoscope twice or maybe three times, did one internal exam, chatted reassuringly, and brought Zak and me some hospital food for dinner, which we ate ravenously except for the succotash.

The pads under Loretta on the labor bed periodically were removed with more bloody show on them. This, I came to understand, was a series of signs of the progress of labor. (Bloody show, recall, is the passing of the mucous plug which has helped seal off the cervix for nine months; when the cervix begins to open up, and continues to open up, this plug slips out.) At one point the nurse mentioned that an increase in the show would indicate the final moments of transition, that is, the finishing up of the dilatation task and the beginning of the expulsion task.

When we arrived at the hospital, Dr. Kurtz had found Loretta to be dilated already 5 cm. He was surprised at the extent of dilatation, given the mild quality of the contractions. The diarrhea must have helped, he suggested, and he wasn't kidding.

From 5 cm to 10 cm we chatted between timing of the contractions. When the relaxed breathing didn't work anymore, Loretta began panting.

Back pain bothered Loretta after every contraction. The baby was probably posterior at this point. The deep, slow breathing (they called it "effacement breathing") was working well to distract from and counteract the pain of contraction, but the backache was another story. A sandbag offered by the nurse, a hard small pillow to wedge against the painful part of the back, was immediately successful as a remedy. The nurse encouraged Loretta to make regular trips to the bathroom. We all breathed with her.

The nurse offered 50 mg of Demerol. Zak and I later agreed that the offer had seemed quite inappropriate—so early in labor, and Loretta clearly managing well. But the nurse hadn't come to know Loretta yet. There were no other offers, nor any requests, but for one time, near end of transition, when Loretta croaked out that this would be the time for drugs; I reminded her it was so near pushing that there really wasn't a point; we just tossed the idea away, and it never returned.

Around 6:00, Loretta threw in a few blows with the panting. Contractions had reached a new level of intensity, her breathing was informing her. She began using an 8-8 pattern, 8 pants, and 8 blows in rhythm. The nurse checked at this point and said that dilating was close to complete, with just an anterior lip of the cervix left. This was overenthusiastic, it turned out.

Dr. Kurtz came in and did an exam during a contraction, and told us the baby's head was in fact transverse (not the whole baby, just the head). He put Loretta on her side to encourage the baby to shift appropriately, and then we had some more transition. For Loretta, lying that way was not as comfortable as being semi-upright on her back. But it worked just right. The doctor manually pushed back the last bit of cervix.

We might as well have been at home, really. Afternoon became evening, we could see trees and lights in the city. The nurse would stop in, make a suggestion or two, give encouragement, and then slip away. Dr. Kurtz was in and out a few times, smiling, with quiet conversation. Everyone acted as if it was altogether natural that I was there, which it was, though somehow one does not expect that sort of welcome in a hospital.

It's hard to get accustomed to pushing. All the learning you've just been acting out, relaxing and rising above the contractions of transition, holding firmly to a pant-blow rhythm, sometimes having to resist the dire urge to push—all that is suddenly no longer relevant to the task at hand, pushing the baby out.

Loretta felt a lot of discomfort after pushing through a contraction, pain in vagina, pain in belly, pain in back. Dr. Kurtz told her that she would feel as if she were splitting apart, but that she wasn't going to split apart. Zak and I gave Loretta water, wiped her face, tried some back massage. Throughout was Loretta's graciousness and her apologies to us all for making a fuss when something would hurt.

Then we organized the pushing effort, with Zak on one side of Loretta and me on the other, pulling up Loretta's knees and coaching the pushing. The nurse put up the sides of the bed, to brace our lady's feet on. We could see the patch of baby's dark hair, advancing and receding with the pushes. Second-stage contractions are farther apart than first-stage; it was smart to learn to relax right away in between them, to get some much-needed rest.

The fetal heart monitor machine sat like a stereo unnoticed in the corner of the room. In this hospital birth there was no bustle, no interference to brace against. Although she was a fine companion in labor, the nurse chose mostly not to stay with us, I guess because it was obvious that we three were doing well together.

Soon we were rolling quietly down the corridor to the delivery room. There was no medical drama being played out here.

Once we got to the delivery room, the nurse quickly prepared, putting Loretta's legs into stirrups and taking her blood pressure.

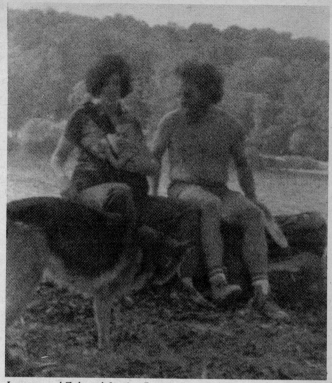

Loretta and Zak and Jessica Rose.

Loretta was settled comfortably on the right spot on the delivery table, washed, draped, shown the hand-holds. When a contraction would come, she would push, and we would cheer. Then the nurse would attend to other preparations, arranging the suturing tools, getting the birth papers together, etc. The pushing continued, and the patch of hair pressed forward, no longer sliding back. Soon it was time to get injected with a local anesthetic for the perineal cut. (When we were suiting up to move from labor to delivery, the doctor had come in and said, "Now, have we spoken about episiotomy?" And Loretta had replied, with a slight groan, "Oh, just do it," and we all laughed.)

The big needle jabbed into the perineum. We all watched the mirror: the scissor snipped and the blood came gushing (this was hard for me to watch).

Dr. Kurtz's instruction: "Now, Loretta, this time I'll tell you to pant," which he did. And she did.

And the head just slid right out, tiny and purplish. Loretta gave a little push for the shoulders, and then a remarkable moment—a cry, a baby with arms and hands and ears and a head now using its own voice, and we were all seeing and hearing the baby, and we didn't even know yet whether it was Jonathan or Jessica.

Then gush and slide, the baby's out, it's Jessica for sure, 8:26 P.M., and she's down on the sterile drape on her mother's belly—all *four* of us amazed as we watched this tiny, yelling 7-pound 6-ounce person turn pink before our eyes.

Dr. Kurtz clamped and cut the cord, after some pulsing, and gave a couple of tugs on the cord, but the placenta wasn't ready. He did some suturing, then tugged again. Finally, a few minutes later, the placenta did come out (I was looking at the baby at the time, noticing how blue her eyes were, so I didn't witness the afterbirth). After footprints and eyedrops for the baby, we propped Loretta up and she put her nipple to her baby's mouth. And suck she did, Jessica Rose.

HOME BIRTH

"All prospective parents should recognize that birth is a critical moment for both mother and child. It is impossible to eliminate *all* risk. Home birth presents one set of risks, mostly connected with the absence of emergency equipment. . . . Hospital birth presents another set of risks, mostly connected with unwarranted intervention. . . . Ultimately a couple must decide, on the basis of personal feelings and values, what's most important to them" (*Woman's Day*, June 28, 1977).

Margaret Mead: ". . . natural childbirth has been a valuable corrective for too much emphasis on pain and anesthesia for the avoidance of pain, and too much emphasis on medical convenience and efficiency, appropriate for hazardous cases, but sometimes an impediment to ordinary births" (*Pregnancy, Birth & the Newborn Baby*).

Between 1972 and 1975, when the overall birth rate on this continent showed a decline, there was a 60% increase in reported out-of-hospital birth. The overwhelming majority of these were home births.

The National Center for Health Statistics reports a 51% increase between 1974 and 1975 in out-of-hospital births.

General features: benefits and risks

In January of 1976 the American College of Obstetricians and Gyne-cologists (ACOG) released a position paper on home birth, conclud-ing that only hospitals can supply appropriate safeguards. "Labor and delivery, while a physiological process, clearly presents potential hazards to both mother and fetus before and after birth. These hazards require standards of safety which are provided in the hospital setting and cannot be matched in the home situation." ACOG was quoting from the *Woman's Day* home-birth article cited above. Canadian doctors, reports Fredelle Maynard in that article, tend to agree.

A majority of childbearing couples, undoubtedly, also agree with the cautions in this recommendation. Even with careful prenatal screening, and even assuming, as does Dr. James Brew (home-birth-oriented obstetrician around Washington, D.C.) that "dangerous deliveries are almost all predictable," women laboring at home do sometimes develop emergency conditions, threatening the baby and/or themselves. Approximately 10% of home-birth mothers in the U.S. end up delivering in hospital because of complications during labor.

"How great is the probability that something may go wrong during a home birth?" writes Marion Sousa in *Childbirth at Home*. "One physician I queried said that for a woman with a history of previously normal births, who is well motivated and receives good prenatal care, the risks are less than one percent."

No one advocates unattended home birth. Couples have successfully navigated such a course, but the risks are sharply increased without knowledgeable outside help and advice.

To find an attendant who will come to your home for your birthing, the best thing to do is to ask around. Obviously ACHI (Association for Childbirth at Home, International) can help (see Chapter 6). CEA (Childbirth Education Association) can help too. And if there are any nurse-midwives in your area, ask them.

Tonya Brooks of ACHI, based in California where the home-birth movement has the most numerous and vocal adherents, suggests that finding an attendant can be tricky. Doctors, after all, even if they support home birth themselves, may lose hospital privileges or insur-ance or both if they attend at home birth. Nurse-midwives, a natural choice, are barred by licensing from attending at home without a physician present. Lay midwives, who if they practice without a physician are practicing illegally, can be hard to locate.

There are women, too, whose credentials as midwives do not yet inspire confidence to entrust one's birthing experience to them. Tonya

Brooks suggests that you draw up an informal checklist for yourself, including such items as:

—What can she handle?
—What is her experience?
—How does she manage third stage?
—Does she suture?
—What does she do in case of hemorrhage?

The statistics which are accumulating from home birth will look even better, suggests Brooks, when medical backup gets more serious and organized.

The level of responsibility that a couple takes upon themselves in electing to give birth at home is great enough in our society to scare away many who support the idea of home birth and would like to experience its benefits.

Parents whose home birth has a less than successful outcome are usually in for some blame from society, unlike parents who have given over management of the birth experience to an institution and suffer a similar outcome. Once again, home birth represents a greater assumption of responsibility by parents. Parents of an infant born at home who dies may be prosecuted for negligence.

Concrete risks include: prolapsed cord, fetal distress, abruption of the placenta, hemorrhage, dysfunctional (no progress) labor.

When birth takes place away from a hospital, there is the crucial question of medical back-up: how far is the home (or maternity center) from emergency medical help? The English have "flying squads," which sounds romantic, but is essentially very sound. A district midwife attending the laboring woman would have a well-equipped ambulance stationed at the nearest hospital, ready to come out with an obstetrician and full emergency equipment if the midwife called for help.

All responsible attendants of home birth work out contingency plans during prenatal preparation. Still, given the risks and acknowledged unknowns, more and more childbearing couples are deciding to stay home. As we will see, it's usually much less expensive than any other option. But that is not its whole appeal.

To maximize the safety and minimize the risk, responsible advocacy groups and facilities who regularly attend or support home birth have developed stringent screening procedures. NAPSAC reports on such procedures in use in the Washington, D.C., area, where a birth center known as Maternity Center Associates (not to be confused with MCA in New York) has been doing home births since October, 1975. This group has medical and nonmedical criteria.

Nonmedical criteria include:

- 10 miles or less from hospital
- willingness to transport self and/or infant to hospital if nurse-midwife or physician thinks it is necessary
- locating a pediatrician who will see baby within 24 hours of birth
- attending childbirth preparation classes
- agreeing to make preparations at home

Medically, the client must have *no* evidence of:

- hypertension, epilepsy, active syphilis or tuberculosis, Rh problem, severe anemia, severe psychiatric distress, diabetes, heart or kidney disease
- multiple birth, pre-eclampsia, abnormal vaginal bleeding, unusual presentation of fetus, previous Caesarean section

Furthermore, the client must be between 15 and 42, have four or fewer children, and be checked for cephalopelvic disproportion.

This set of criteria is clearly stringent enough to sort out the risk population from the 90% or so of us who can expect by natural selection to give birth without complication. ACHI, the largest, most active home-birth organization (teachers and trainees now number over 200, and groups exist in 38 states), is similarly cautious in describing the appropriate low-risk candidate for home birth. Along with such criteria as those listed above, they require a standard of health outside the normal medical definition, including good vitality and muscle tone.

Medical benefits of home birth include less risk of infection than in the hospital (contrary to what hospitals would have us believe). Marshall Klaus, drawing from recent findings in endocrinology, ethology, infant development, immunology, and bacteriology, points to the lower risks involved when the baby's bacteria are "colonized with the mother's rather than with the hospital's bacteria." Dr. Gregory White agrees: the baby born at home has the benefit of not being sneezed on or handled by the many people a hospital environment accommodates, of being born in a place where nobody was born earlier that day.

The relationship between postpartum depression and place of birth is worth taking note of. Postpartum depression, an effect of amazing regularity in the lore of childbirth, awaits research findings and analysis from the social sciences before we can adequately characterize or treat it. Tonya Brooks of ACHI has figures of her own that put the incidence of this depression at about 65% of women; for 20% of these it is severe enough to be labeled psychosis, and 2% of these do not recover. The manner of our birthing, concludes Tonya, has far-reaching effects on our emotional state.

Raven Lang quotes a California physician as having observed a noticeably lower incidence of postpartum depression in home-birth mothers than in hospital-birth mothers.

Lang's observation consolidates and supports preliminary theories of Klaus and others regarding what they call disorders of mothering, interruptions in the building of the essential bond between mother and infant. In *Childbirth at Home,* Marion Sousa reports this effect: "Several studies have shown that premature babies who had to be separated from their mothers and specially cared for during their first few weeks of life may later suffer terrible consequences. Between 25% and 40% of our battered children have spent their first few weeks of life in a nursery for premature infants. Apparently, after the immediate separation following birth, their mothers were simply unable to form the normal emotional bonds with their babies."

The primary reported benefit from giving birth at home is the opportunity to stay together in a familiar atmosphere: not to be separated, mother and child from each other, family members from the newborn. The normal hospital procedure of removing infants to the nursery for up to 24 hours before reuniting mother and child is seen by home-birth proponents as a *deprivation* of inherent biological *rights* of parent(s) and offspring.

One mother made a comparison for Fredelle Maynard in the *Woman's Day* article cited at the beginning of this chapter:

> When Miriam was born in the hospital, the nurse held her up and said, "You've got a lovely girl—ten fingers, ten toes." Then she whisked her away. When Matthew was born at home, I sat up all night looking at him, touching and smelling. The most tremendous love and tenderness came over me that night. I still feel it—and it's spilled over to Miriam.

With home birth, too, other children in the family can come to bond with the newcomer, can understand the organic addition to their family unit in a way that a hospital situation prevents them from being able to.

Lewis Mehl, Director of the NAPSAC Childbirth Research Institute, is one of the most outspoken doctors regarding the value of home birth. In a study reported to the 104th annual meeting of the American Public Health Association in October, 1976, he used matched populations to compare outcomes for hospital-birth and home-birth parents. Given data from countries like the Netherlands, and given the kind of "psycho-social advantages proposed by advocates of home delivery," he asks, mildly enough, ". . . is it possible that under some conditions home delivery may be a reasonable alternative in the United States?" To test his question he matched two populations—

·1046 who delivered at home, 1046 who delivered at a hospital—according to maternal age, number of previous children, socioeconomic status, and prenatal medical condition.

The hospital births featured more oxytocin before and after delivery, and it was administered intravenously; when home-birth mothers received the hormone, in cases of dysfunction, it was given by mouth and in lesser dosages. Home births took longer. Also, Mehl noted greater use or greater occurrence of the following in hospital births: forceps, Caesarean section, episiotomy, perineal tear, analgesia, anesthesia, fetal distress, hypertension, meconium staining, postpartum maternal hemmorhage, birth injury, fetal infection, resuscitation, and lower Apgar scores.

In addition, attendants at hospital births turned to forceps after an hour of second stage; the home-birth attendants used a different standard, using forceps only when there was a lack of progress in the labor. Interference in posterior labor did not tend to occur in the home births, but did, with the use of forceps, in the hospital.

Sources of information and support

There are good books to consult if you have an interest in home birth. NAPSAC has collected articles from doctors, parents, and midwives on the topic *Safe Alternatives in Childbirth*; the publication is based on their first conference in May of 1976. A similar conference was convened in March of 1977, and the proceedings (*21st-Century Obstetrics Now*) from that are due to be published soon.

The 1976 NAPSAC anthology, winner of the Books of the Year Award from the *American Journal of Nursing*, was edited by David and Lee Stewart. Its table of contents gives an idea of the range of what some of our leading childbirth educators consider to be safe alternatives: the viability of the home-birth option is suggested in some of the titles:

HOMEBIRTHS—A MODERN TREND—IS IT PROGRESS?
by David Stewart

WHY IS THERE A NEED FOR ALTERNATIVES IN CHILDBIRTH?
by Lee Stewart

MATERNITY PRACTICES AROUND THE WORLD: HOW DO WE MEASURE UP?
by Doris Haire

CHILDBEARING & MATERNITY CENTERS: ALTERNATIVES TO HOMEBIRTH AND HOSPITAL
by Betty Hosford and Ruth Watson Lubic

CHILDBIRTH ALTERNATIVES & INFANT OUTCOME: A PEDIATRIC VIEW
  by Robert Mendelsohn

COMPARATIVE STUDY OF OBSTETRICS—WITH DATA & DETAILS OF A
  WORKING PHYSICIAN'S OB SERVICE
    by Frederic M. Ettner

HOMEBIRTHS AND THE PHYSICIAN
  by Mayer Eisentein

STATISTICAL OUTCOMES OF HOMEBIRTHS IN THE UNITED STATES:
  CURRENT STATUS
    by Lewis E. Mehl

BIRTH-RELATED MORTALITY RATES BY SIZE & TYPE OF HOSPITAL
  by Doris Haire

A SAFE HOMEBIRTH PROGRAM THAT WORKS
  by Janet L. Epstein, James D. Brew, et al.

THE LAY MIDWIFE
  by Nancy Mills

WHY DO RESPONSIBLE, INFORMED PARENTS CHOOSE HOMEBIRTHS?
  (Four essays by parents opting for birth at home)

LEGAL ASPECTS OF HOMEBIRTH & OTHER CHILDBIRTH ALTERNATIVES
  by George J. Annas

Across the top of the back cover of the book runs the following statement by NAPSAC: "Hospitals have never been proven to be the safest place for most mothers to give birth to their babies."

Fred Ward and Charlotte Ward have produced *The Home Birth Book,* a collection of documents, data, reflections, and personal experiences. This one includes some marvelous photographs. It is especially illuminating, in both this and the NAPSAC, to read commentary by physicians, because they are the ones who will close the gap, or rather, help strengthen the bridges built over it. Dr. James Brew, obstetrician who attends home births in the Washington, D.C., area, points out: "To fully realize the significance of home-birth, I think it is necessary to look honestly at the tangible benefits to the new baby. . . . First, and most important, the new baby is kept in the family where it belongs." The book contains writings about the psychological dimension of home birth ("On Imprinting" by midwife Raven Lang), numerous profiles of home-birth families, and practical directions for more reading and for needed supplies and preparations.

Marion Sousa's *Childbirth at Home,* to which we have already referred, is packed with practical advice and theoretical/statistical background. Sousa delves into such difficult areas as resuscitation of a greatly damaged baby. She describes hospital birth, and includes many personal narratives.

In *Mother Love,* a book devoted mainly to the art of childrearing, Alice Bricklin describes the home birth of her third child and makes the suggestion, heard widely, that nurse-midwives would be an excellent source of attendants for the growing number of families who wish to share the birth of a baby in their own home.

Of the manuals available for emergency birth, the best known is Dr. Gergory White's *Emergency Childbirth,* strongly recommended by most educators on the subject. The Association for Childbirth at Home, International (ACHI, formerly ACAH) has also published an informative manual, called *Giving Birth at Home,* available directly from the California headquarters (see Chapter 6 for address). ACHI will be reissuing the manual with some revisions soon.

Raven Lang's *Birth Book* is a classic by now. In this one, remarkable photos and first-person stories combine with a historically-oriented introduction.

Popular media have been investigating the phenomenon of home birth as it has been growing. Of the many popular magazine articles, one of the most notable is the one from *Woman's Day* (June 28, 1977) quoted at the beginning of this chapter. By Fredelle Maynard, the article, called "Home Birth vs. Hospital Birth," describes the issues clearly and with good backup information.

In the NAPSAC chapter "Statistical Outcomes of Homebirths in the U.S.: Current Status," Dr. Lewis Mehl summarizes prevalent attitudes in his profession:

> Generally, the response of physicians to home delivery has been negative. Many view homebirth as an irresponsible risk to mother and child. They do not encourage or attend home deliveries, and many have refused to give prenatal care, advice or instruction to couples planning homebirth. A dichotomy exists in obstetrics today between the technological trend represented by high risk obstetric units with fetal monitoring and readily available medical and surgical intervention, and the family-centered, natural childbirth trend represented in its extreme by couples planning home delivery *without medical support*. We feel that reducing the antagonism between these divergent poles would enhance care of women choosing hospital as well as home deliveries.

The dichotomy to which Dr. Mehl refers is the subject of a recent paper by Ruth Lubic, "Fetal Electronic Monitoring Vs. Home Delivery," based on her address to the Twenty-Fifth Annual National

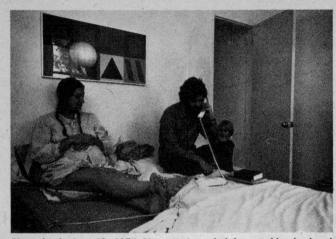

Home birth, June 12, 1974. Nancy is in early labor, and her husband Alvin is calling the midwife. The child in the doorway is a neighbor child.

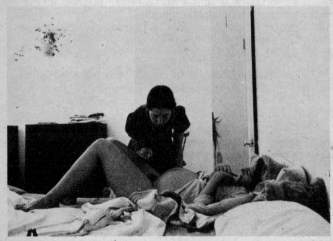

Midwife Lisa checks the fetal heartbeat. Lisa began her midwife career in Italy at the age of 13, when she accompanied a neighbor to a birthing in an emergency.

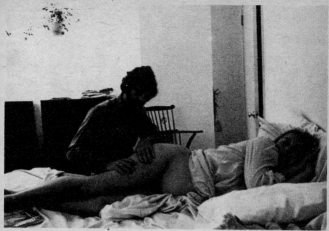

Cramps and muscle tightening are not uncommon; here her husband is able to help Nancy become more comfortable as labor progresses by giving a massage.

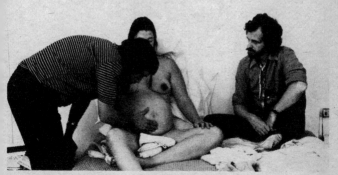

Dr. John Carpenter has arrived and is checking the baby's position. Nancy, in active labor, is more comfortable without her gown.

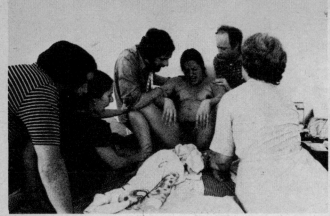

Second stage labor. Nancy is supported by her husband and by the midwife's husband. Other supporters are the doctor, the midwife, and the midwife's mother. Nancy's own mother was also present. The baby is about to appear.

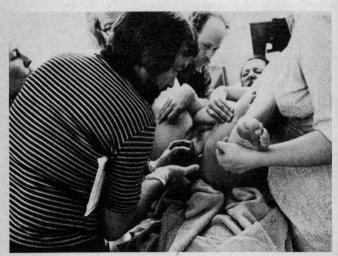

The baby's head is now crowning, and Dr. Carpenter is ready to catch.

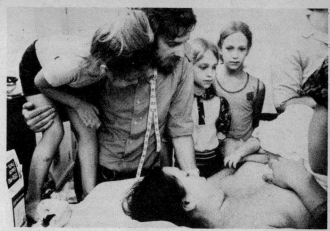

Neighbor children and the couple's daughter Alice watch just-born Elizabeth as she takes her first looks around and her first sucks. Alvin wears a tape measure to find out the length of his new daughter.

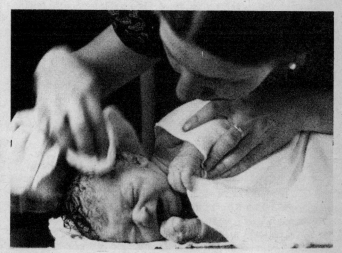

Elizabeth gets wiped off by Lisa. Birthday cake and champagne followed.

Health Forum, March 23, 1977. In this consumer-oriented approach, Lubic characterizes the polarization in maternity care today by opposing fetal monitoring (symbolic of high-risk obstetric technology) on the one hand with home delivery (low-risk family-centered care) on the other. Home delivery, she notes, is increasingly becoming the choice of childbearing couples even when a qualified attendant cannot be found. Yet, as data from the two poles are not conclusive, Lubic urges a compromise position whereby care that is acceptable both to consumers and to obstetric personnel be made available. Lubic points to the idea of the maternity center as a reasonable middle ground.

For Judy Norsigian of *Our Bodies, Ourselves*, the polarity between hospital and home birth is, among other things, the basis for the issue of the right to choose. In an unpublished paper (1977) entitled "Out-of-Hospital Birth," Norsigian comments thus: "In most situations when a complication arises, there is ample time to reach a hospital before there is any great threat to either mother or baby. However, it *is* true that there are risks to out-of-hospital birth, just as there are risks to in-hospital birth. The important issue here is not to prove that one setting is necessarily better than another, but to point out that a controversy exists and that parents have the right to decide for themselves which risks they want to take when choosing where and how they want to give birth."

Nonmedically speaking, then, besides being able to keep the family together for a peak experience, the other major benefit for most couples of having birth at home is the element of control. So many women feel helpless in hospital-birth situations, robbed of their dignity, treated like children, or as cases, practiced upon, strapped down, yanked on, delivered of. The overwhelming reaction of home-birth parents is that they truly *gave* birth, that they participated meaningfully in the management of this most remarkable event in their lives.

Sue and Jonah did it this way.

Story: Sue and Jonah

Sue and Jonah gave birth to their first child one day late in May in their West Philadelphia apartment. They are good neighbors and new friends; I began to know them during Sue's pregnancy. Although I was not present on Kate's birthday, I feel close to their story.

Their decision to have a home birth developed gradually. Once Sue discovered she was pregnant, she and Jonah began going to Booth Maternity Center. Both felt good about the prenatal care they were receiving, and liked the facilities at Booth, but neither was happy at heart with anything at all like a hospital. Jonah, 24, is a yoga and massage teacher; Sue, 20, is a specialist in nutrition and herbs. Both are vegetarians. They began to want to investigate the possibility of having their baby at home. Inquiries revealed that in all of Philadelphia only one obstetrician was available to attend home deliveries, Dr. John Carpenter. Sue and Jonah located him, visited him, and, at about 5½ months pregnant, set about planning for their home birth.

Dr. Carpenter, pictured in the home photo sequence above (*not* Sue and Jonah's) in this chapter, has been attending home births for about seven years, accompanied by a lay midwife. In his view the statistics on home birth are good and the chance of sudden emergency is rare; he believes that most obstetricians are not willing to undertake home birth because scheduling and lack of backup cause inconvenience in the doctor's life, because it takes more effort, because they worry about malpractice, and because they are not convinced it is safe. (Dr. Carpenter will be working primarily with a new home-birth style unit at a local hospital as soon as the facility gets final approval.)

Betsy, the lay midwife who has frequently accompanied Dr. Carpenter, has been working around Philadelphia for four years. She has assisted at the delivery of several dozen babies. Most of Sue's prenatal care was in the hands of Dr. Carpenter, but about two weeks before the baby was due Betsy visited with Sue and Jonah at their apartment to discuss arrangements for the birth. Betsy explained the necessary preparations, including a car with a full tank of gas ready to go to the hospital, ten minutes away. She also explained that if Sue's hemoglobin count were to drop below 12, home birth would be ruled out because of the extra risk attendant upon a low count. (Hemoglobin, which comes to us from iron, absorbs oxygen from the mother's lungs and carries it to the mother's tissues and to the baby; the normal range is 11.6 to 14.)

Betsy sometimes works alone, too—that is, without Dr. Carpenter. She is friendly with nurse-midwives in the area, and it is my impression that among them there is much mutual sympathy.

As the pregnancy progressed, and Sue's health remained fine, she and Jonah began to think they would not need to call on Dr. Carpenter at all; since Betsy was (is) comfortable attending deliveries unassisted when there is no sign of complication, it seemed like a possible development. But, Sue said, when she had her last prenatal visit with Dr. Carpenter and told him they were thinking of managing without him, his response was that he wanted to be there, that it wouldn't be a problem for him at all. And so they revised the plan. Sue now says she was glad he attended, even though there were no medical problems.

Sue and Jonah had planned to invite some friends for the birth. Eight-year-old Rebecca and several taller people were looking forward to being there to see the baby come out. But when the time came, Sue and Jonah didn't call anyone. There is a limit to the amount of diffusion of attention one can handle during labor; their instincts told them they had enough to concentrate on.

To return to chronology. Sue and Jonah's prenatal preparation included classes with Marie Larello, the well known Lamaze instructor with whom Zak and Loretta also had prepared. Sue attended a lecture given by Tonya Brooks, founder of ACHI, and was inspired to want to take the six-class series offered by the Association; but with the Lamaze classes and her own work (which she continued right up to the end), it was not practical.

Sue talked about the amazing learning that the experience of labor gives. The effort to stay in control, to not lose her grip, during what turned out to be a long first stage, the excitement of pushing all out in second stage, somehow these experiences were showing her parts of herself that were new. And how personal every labor is! Your own body, doing a giant task it was designed for, can tell you about yourself if you stay in the ring with it, stay aware, watch yourself through all. Sue laughed and gestured toward the ceiling; saying it was as if she were up there, in the corner of the room, looking down upon herself as she waited out those hours of dilatation. And then, when called upon, she jumped right in to do the pushing.

I asked Jonah and Sue if they had felt afraid of the risks in home birth. They had, Sue said, given it a lot of thought. The precautions of the doctor were reassuring, and even more so was Betsy's careful attitude. Midwives traditionally use conservative criteria for deciding when to ask for help; they are in no way burdened with pride about holding off in going to the hospital, or about asking for advice and help. They do not want to undertake more than they are capable of handling. (Tonya Brooks: "We would all rather see ten women who didn't really need to, go to the hospital than see one who should, not go.") Even with such an attitude, there are scares. Betsy had only recently attended at a birth which was uncomplicated until after the delivery of the placenta, when the woman began suddenly to hemorrhage. She was saved, after a quick ride to a nearby hospital, but there is a terrible fright in such a turn of events.

Yes, there are risks in home birth. One in 200 labors is complicated by cord prolapse, for example, not the sort of predictable occurrence that, say, breech position usually is. But the arrangements and the proximity of the University Hospital were, for Jonah and Sue, reasonable insurance against disaster. And, as they pointed out, there are risks, no matter where you go. At some point, having done your best, you put your trust in God and in your own ability.

For Sue there were a couple of days of painless, but noticeable, contractions before labor actually began. During this period she was also passing mucus, often blood-flecked, an example of an extended ''show.''

At one o'clock in the morning that day in May, Sue began needing to breathe consciously to stay on top of the contractions; at 5:00 A.M., with contractions coming every 3 minutes or so, they called Betsy, who arrived a half hour later. There followed the standard exam: blood pressure; fetal heart rate; internal examination, revealing that Sue's cervix was open to 5 cm; and the midwife's usual advice, to get up, move around, urinate.

Sue knew that dilatation might take some time. At her last checkup Dr. Carpenter had noted that she had a tight cervix. Women vary widely in the elasticity of their cervix before labor begins. If a woman's cervix is flexible, labor may be quite short.

As often happens, the arrival of the midwife brought a temporary lull to the progress of the contractions. Many women experience this kind of slowdown when they leave the security and familiarity of their home to take the trip, however short and smooth, to the hospital, and get checked in, prepared, and settled in the labor bed. At Betsy's suggestion, Sue and Jonah went out for a walk at 7:00 that morning to stimulate the labor and clear their heads. Jonah later remarked to me about the value of a change like that walk—when the atmosphere in the one same room begins to feel stale, a change can blow things clear again. Sure enough, contractions revived as they moved slowly through the early morning activity of the neighborhood. As they sat by the door of a local ashram, Sue's water broke, and, simultaneously, morning chanting began.

And so, for all that day, Sue labored. She felt powerful discomfort in her lower back and pubic bone area, and the pain did not altogether subside at the end of each contraction. This was a posterior labor—the back of the baby's head was resting against the mother's back, giving that characteristic ''back labor'' kind of pain. As labor progressed, slowly, the apprentice midwife who accompanied Betsy applied warm towels to Sue's abdomen—a great help, she says.

Sue didn't feel like eating, after a peach or two early in the morning. In her herbal studies Sue learned about tinctures from various flowers and plants which can be combined to provide medicinal help in various physical situations, and a tincture to be used in a time of stress was the only ''nourishment'' she took during the day.

By early afternoon, Sue was discouraged to find herself only 7 cm dilated. With the membranes ruptured, she was concerned about the battering of the baby's head against the bones around the cervix. Betsy was able to reassure her, encourage, sympathize, and bolster her spirits. Yet when Dr. Carpenter arrived around 6:30 in the evening, he found the dilatation still to be less than 8 cm. This was another setback for Sue's occasionally floundering spirits.

As Dr. Carpenter stood by the bed with Betsy discussing the dilatation, Jonah, empathetic with Sue and also feeling a break in concentration, asked the doctor and the midwife to leave the room. They promptly and agreeably did, had some watermelon, compared notes, and soon returned to the business at hand. Sue and Jonah got the time they needed alone and were grateful for the sensitivity that made that request from them easily accepted by the professional attendants.

The doctor was able manually to "get rid of" the last bit of cervix, that is, push back the part of the rim still present, saving Sue probably another hour or so of transition. The first stage was now over.

Able at last to push, Sue got right into it. Second stage for her was very short. By this time the baby had turned the 180 degrees necessary to present in the usual anterior way—that is, face down, which insures a much smoother descent through the birth canal. The head began to crown after just a few pushes, and one of the midwives showed Sue that she could touch the head there at the vaginal opening. What a remarkable feeling *that* must be!

In a hospital, of course, the woman must keep her hands away from her perineum. She is not permitted even to touch the drape over her abdomen; she is kept thoroughly separated from the action, except for a view from the overhead mirror. (As Sue and many home-birth advocates have pointed out, a baby born at home amid reasonable cleanliness is relatively safe from strong foreign infections. In "antiseptic" hospital nurseries, staph infections are a constant threat. At home, the germs are the baby's own, anyway. Of course, Betsy's prenatal instruction had included sterilizing some basic items; and she spread a sterile cloth on the bed for second stage—which, in most instances, is cleanliness aplenty.)

Betsy and Dr. Carpenter coached Sue carefully to keep the baby's emergence slow and smooth. Everyone there, Sue later recalled, was busy and appreciated. She was doing the pushing, the apprentice midwife and Jonah were holding her up, Betsy was giving encouragement, Dr. Carpenter was ready to catch, and Kate was moving rapidly down the birth canal. Though her cervix had been tight and slow to open, Sue's perineum had considerable elasticity. The doctor and midwife both helped to stretch it out with their fingers, and the head was born with no cuts or lacerations. Like most undrugged babies, this one began to cry then, only partly born.

The shoulders emerged somewhat abruptly, causing a tear small enough to be closed up with one stitch. Then Kate was out, 8:40 P.M., and was right then put on her naked mother's abdomen.

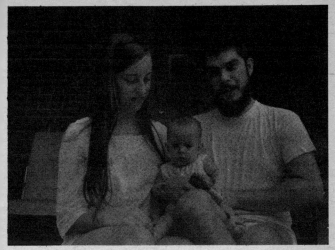

Sue and Jonah and Kate.

Sue and Jonah felt the cord as it pulsed its last; then it was cut. The placenta emerged without difficulty. (The next morning, Sue added a bit of placenta to some vegetable juice with raw egg and drank the mixture.)

Kate was put to breast but, busy with vigorous crying, was not interested for the moment. Sue got up and took a bath while Betsy sat with her and answered questions. Jonah, meanwhile, bathed his tiny daughter in warm water. The three slept together in the big bed.

THE IDEA OF THE MATERNITY CENTER

There is a kind of facility which in some ways is like a hospital and in some ways is not like a hospital. It is friendly in ways that a home is, though it is not anyone's home. It can be found in many places, this kind of obstetrical facility: in the middle of a large hospital on New York City's Upper West Side; in a brownstone dwelling, basement floor, a few blocks away from there; in a Salvation Army hospital for pregnant single teenagers on the Philadelphia suburban line; in an old dispensary building in a run-down section of Chicago; amid the greenery and hospitality of a small northwest city. You name it, there could be a maternity center there.

In this section we will describe the idea of the maternity center and take a look at some examples, both in hospital and out.

Maternity centers appeal to consumers, to childbearing couples. They are often staffed by nurse-midwives. They specialize in low-risk obstetrical cases. Intellectually, they often look to the theoretical/empirical work of doctors like Klaus in the United States, and Bowlby in England, to keep their childbearing programs apace with the most important academic findings of their research colleagues. One could characterize their medical standards as generally conservative: that is, they do not push their luck, they are not looking for fast, flashy results. The collection of data in the area of maternity-center birth, as in the area of home birth, is careful. Maternity centers seek to know their clientele; their services cost a reasonable amount, they emphasize continuity of care, and they hold family life to be a primary value.

Dr. Lewis Mehl summarizes his comparison of home-birth and hospital-birth outcomes this way: "It . . . seems appropriate to conclude that for low medical risk women, home delivery is an alternative that cannot be dismissed. . . . From these results it would seem reasonable and prudent to plan pilot projects in out-of-hospital deliveries or in changing hospital policy to create a more home-like environment."

Dr. Klaus, pediatrician and theorist, imagines a similar possibility in *Maternal-Infant Bonding:* "Ideally, we would like to use the best of present day knowledge of high-risk obstetrics, neonatology, infant development, and mother-infant attachment and at the same time have family and parent participation in homelike births in the hospital."

The maternity center offers this kind of obstetrical care in hospital and out.

Kitty Ernst of Maternity Center Association (MCA) in New York believes there is room for a maternity center every ten blocks in the city. With good medical backup and the eagle-eyed screening procedures which MCA (among others) insists upon, such community facilities could provide a safe, inexpensive, and pleasant atmosphere for normal births.

It's not such a new idea, the maternity center. In Europe they have existed for centuries. In this country and Canada, freestanding maternity centers are now opening up in communities of every size. Oklahoma City has a new one; Eugene (Oregon) and Albuquerque (New Mexico) have had maternity centers since about the time MCA opened its Childbearing Center (autumn, 1975). MCA serves as unofficial coordinator and dispenser of information about this kind of facility.

Booth Maternity Center in Philadelphia differs from these in being an actual hospital, equipped for surgery, and licensed as a hospital. And hospitals themselves are beginning to open up special facilities within their walls that cater specifically to the population which wants prepared, low-medication, family-centered, "natural," home-like birth.

Flower-Fifth Avenue Hospital (defunct as of 1978) in the Upper West Side of New York City was an example of a large, university-related hospital in which a home-like birthing place had been made available. Rather like a special zone, this facility used to operate amidst the kinds of conditions which it was designed to contrast with. Dr. Don Sloan is a New York obstetrician who teamed up with Elisabeth Bing, the noted childbirth educator and co-founder of the Lamaze organization in this country, to develop the program at Flower-Fifth Avenue. In 1976, Dr. Sloan told me about a recent birthing in which the contrast with the hospital's regular activities was most noticeable; so many of the hospital's services—dietary, pediatrics, nursing—were intersecting there, that he finally had to lock the door from the inside because of the constant coming and going of personnel.

Couples who used this Family-Centered Maternity Program at Flower-Fifth Avenue would take childbirth preparation, such as the Lamaze-style course offered by Ms. Bing and others at the hospital. Dr. Sloan for one, felt strongly that birth is too pathologically viewed in the hospital setting; he was (and is) interested in psychological pain relief. The facility recognized the value of immediate postpartum contact between members of the new family, and actively supported breastfeeding. Labor and delivery would happen in the same bed (which is a fine idea, since the conventional transfer is always awkward at best).

Other hospital-based facilities are beginning to offer a maternity-center style of care. For example, nurse-midwives practice at University Hospital in Minneapolis and at Community Hospital of Springfield and Clark County in Springfield, Ohio. Mt. Zion Hospital in San Francisco has home-like facilities, as does Family Hospital in Milwaukee and Catherine Booth Hospital in Montreal.

McMaster Medical Center in Hamilton, Ontario, and Manchester Memorial Hospital in Connecticut have programs featuring some or most of the "Family-Centered Care" ideas; in the Connecticut facility the particular attraction is European labor-delivery beds and a strong Lamaze orientation. In Fairfield County, Connecticut, the number of "Lamaze deliveries" doubled between 1974 and 1975, from 1200 to 2400.

Hazell shares her fantasies of a Maternity Motel in *Commonsense Childbirth*. With movement in the directions we are now seeing, however, the idea is not nearly so utopian as it seemed six years ago. Establishment of careful, low-risk, family-oriented choices within regular hospitals is a way for those hospitals to stay in touch with what people want, and thus to complete successfully with freestanding maternity centers for business.

Chicago Maternity Center

In its history this facility saw the births of 150,000 people, 90% of them at home. In the 1930s, the peak years of its success, the Chicago Maternity Center (CMC) provided a medical team of a nurse-midwife, student nurse, and two medical students to go out on call. During this decade, when one woman in 400 died from puerperal fever, the CMC lost not a single mother; doing about 3600 births a year, the CMC showed a better record than any area hospital's. Dr. Beatrice Tucker attended or supervised the attendance of a large percentage of these births. Arms quotes her as saying: "I am committed to home births . . . in a hospital, the isolation is devastating."

Begun in 1895 as the Maxwell Street Dispensary by Dr. Joseph B. DeLee, who was horrified at mortality rates (and who, incidentally, introduced forceps in hospital birth), the facility stood for a kind of maternity care we have yet to see on that scale since.

Prenatal care is the key to safe delivery, they felt there; the emphasis was on nutrition and rest.

The Center trained doctors in such skills as how to ask questions, how to help the mother talk about what concerns her, and how to answer her questions. The Center believed that there is "no substitute for the time it takes to give this kind of care," according to the makers of the documentary "The Chicago Maternity Center Story," a 16 mm, 60-minute, black-and-white film made in 1974 by Kartemquin Films, Chicago.

"The Chicago Maternity Center Story" was made with hopes of gathering support for the Center at a time when its existence was being threatened by the controlling medical establishment. Its actual demise occurred when the filming was yet in progress; thus the film contains footage of the decisive confrontations between the CMC community supporters and the hospital administrative board.

Part I of the film is entitled "Health Care Worth Fighting For." It opens with extreme close-up shots of women, not rich, various in background, urgently supporting the Center, urgently in favor of home delivery: birth is natural, they say—it's good for the other kids to see—we would never get such good care anywhere else—we NEED the kind of service this center gives—it's the good, old-fashioned *house call*.

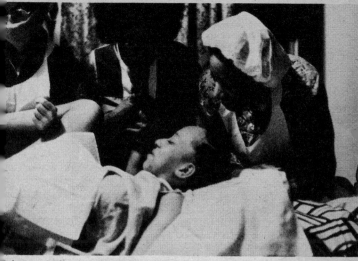

charene Miller in second-stage labor at home, coached by members f her family, attended by Dr. Beatrice Tucker of the Chicago Mater- ity Center.

The film then shows footage of a CMC home birth. Scharene Miller s in labor at home. She is attended by Beatrice Tucker, aged 75, on he staff of CMC for 40 years, its only full-time doctor at the time of he filming.

The mother is definitely uncomfortable, not always in control. Her xtended family is there with her. Delivery is to take place on the lining room table. Masks and gowns and gloves are used. Dr. Tucker, who has been training obstetricians since the 1930s, scrubs he woman's belly. The mother is thrashing and moaning and panting. Dr. Tucker briskly coaches her on breathing (this woman didn't have he money to go to natural childbirth classes). It is a posterior resentation, which means that the baby's descent is less smooth, and abor is more difficult to manage. "The Center staff knows when and low to wait."

Dr. Tucker uses forceps, instructing a young medical student as she loes. It is an exacting, demanding process. Forceps were used in only bout 1% of CMC deliveries, for just this kind of case. Skillfully, ind all the while teaching, Dr. Tucker guides the infant through safe delivery.

Part II of the film, called "The Struggle for Control," documents the Center's losing battle for survival. The kind of care the CMC offered has "no place in the women's health care industry," says a hospital administrator in the film. Of the women then using the center, 45% were black, 40% Latina, 15% white. The cost: up to $50 for all services, for everyone. The center offered comfortable birthing, continuous with the cultural traditions of the clients.

A new women's hospital is now being built in Chicago, at a cost of many millions, supposedly to assume the work of the CMC. It will be staffed by Northwestern University. The filmmakers report how the CMC was to have been relocated inside this new hospital, but Northwestern began withdrawing support from the CMC: "Hospitals are a business," administrators said; and CMC expenses were too much for them to meet.

"We are available for everyone," says the CMC in confrontation with the University board. "The community needs us," says Dr. Tucker. "It is the best care they can receive. It might be their only care." The community rallied support to keep CMC from being wiped out, but the effort was unsuccessful.

The Center was closed by Northwestern Hospital in 1974, at which time studies showed that labor overseen by the CMC had proved to be 8 to 10 times safer than that in the local hospital, Cooke County Hospital. The CMC's closing poses serious consequences for the women of the community whom it once served. Now many of these women, observe the filmmakers, will not see a doctor during their pregnancy at all.

"The Chicago Maternity Center Story" is available for rental as described in Chapter 6. Directors of a program in urban medicine at University of Illinois School of Medicine made this comment: "We shall certainly use this film in our teaching. The Maternity Center is seen not as an outmoded institution, but as an important new model for developing community-based maternity care, compatible with people's economic needs and cultural traditions."

Maternity Center Association

For nearly six years Maternity Center Association in New York has been a guiding light of maternity care and teaching.

As the MCA introductory brochure explains, "In 1918 the United States had the highest maternal death rate of any developed country in the world. Alarmed by this shocking fact, a small group of leading citizens and physicians in New York formed the Maternity Center Association to combat the problem. Today U.S. maternal mortality is among the lowest in the world." (Infant mortality is not such a success story; the U.S. ranks 14th or 15th among industrialized countries.) "Maternity Center continues at the forefront of the struggle to provide equal access to maternity services to raise the quality of care, to erase the deficits in medical man-power."

This work has its headquarters in a large, elegant brownstone in the Upper West Side of New York. There are seven floors of offices and nurse-midwife quarters; in the basement, since late 1975, is the Child-bearing Center, an experiment in low-risk, family-centered, economical maternity care.

There are several major aspects of the work of MCA. In a sense it is the matriarch of maternity centers, committed from the beginning to education, to the work of the nurse-midwife (MCA began the first training of nurse-midwives in 1931), and to development of family-centered maternity care.

Respected worldwide, MCA publishes educational materials in use by parents and professionals throughout this country and in 82 other countries. Foremost among these materials is the *Birth Atlas*, photographs of a series of sculptures exhibited by MCA at the 1939 World's Fair in New York; these life-size sculptures depict the stages of labor. The photographs in Chapter 1 are plates from that series. The *Birth Atlas* is known throughout the world as a symbol of education for childbirth.

MCA has produced films, publishes a regular digest of maternity and child care (*Briefs*), acts as consultant for developing maternity centers, and helps to teach doctors and nurses. As a national and international nonprofit, voluntary, experimental health agency, MCA supports research and development of superior maternity care by testifying before legislatures, guiding government leaders toward the achievement of better national policies for maternal-infant care, sponsoring conferences, giving classes, and acting, at times, the ant, as Kitty Ernst said, to the elephant of Establishment Obstetrics.

MCA's history is colorful, spanning many years and many changes in obstetrics. Some of its milestones are reported in Chapter 4. These include the beginnings of rural maternity nursing services in the mid-1920s, the beginnings of father classes in the 1920s and 1930s, the sponsorship of Dr. Dick-Read's visit in 1947, attendance of home deliveries until the late 1950s, the advancement of nurse-midwifery, aid in the establishment of Booth Maternity Center in 1971, and, in October 1975, the opening of the MCA Childbearing Center.

The MCA Childbearing Center (CbC), like every maternity center facility, is unique. It was designed to offer an atmosphere of pleasant, family-centered maternity care to those who anticipate a normal labor and wish to retain as much control over the childbirth experience as is medically appropriate. In the words of General Director Ruth Lubic,

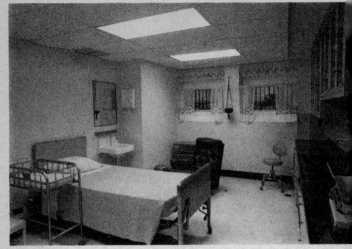

Labor-delivery room at Maternity Center Association's Childbearing Center, New York. The Childbearing Center became active in 1975.

promoting the new MCA facility as a compromise between home-style and hospital-style delivery: "Our Childbearing Center was set up to test whether safe, satisfying and economic care might be provided to a population which was employing do-it-yourself home delivery in blacklash to what they feel is dehumanizing and unsafe hospital care. We seek to provide a sensible, human 'middle ground' to the two trade-off extremes we are examining" (from "Fetal Electronic Monitoring Vs. Home Delivery," based on Lubic's 1977 address to the Twenty-Fifth Annual National Health Forum).

There are two labor-delivery rooms, brightly colored, spacious rooms with plants. With a lounge area and a kitchen, the atmosphere is homelike, reassuring, and comfortable.

The soul of this facility is a staff of nine nurse-midwives who work on rotating shifts. The nurse-midwives provide prenatal education and prenatal care (except for two visits with a doctor), and they attend the couples during labor.

I sat in on a preliminary orientation session at MCA one Saturday afternoon among a group of well-educated, attractive, healthy, and culturally diverse couples. Kitty Ernst, CNM, led the discussion with an emphasis on the value of prenatal care. At the Childbearing Center of MCA, prenatal visits afford an education not only in pregnancy and labor, but also in the physiology of reproduction, in sexuality, the family, oneself, and infant growth and development. The client's chart is anything but a secret.

The program, gradually being phased in to accommodate 500 births a year, is enormously watchful about its medical safety. CbC is not a hospital; a doctor is on hand, or readily available by phone, but the facility is not equipped with fetal heart monitors or surgical potential. In case of hazard or complication, the mother and/or baby are taken to the backup hospital 11 minutes away. No breech or multiple births are delivered at MCA; there is no induction of labor. Intravenous capabilities are part of the equipment, as are "emergency" drugs, infant resuscitation equipment, baby warmers, and oxygen. But the focus is on noninterference.

CbC is not a residential facility. Parents are expected to return home with their baby about 12 hours after the birth. Couples who have tried the program—I met with one young family upstairs in the office—were bubbling with enthusiasm for their MCA childbearing experience.

A $885 fee includes all prenatal care and education, such as the eight-week preparation course ("our version of Lamaze"), and a minimum of two visits with a doctor. Also included are pediatric examination, public health nurse followup at home on the first day and the third or fifth day after birth, and all return visits.

Booth Maternity Center

To the obstetrical establishment, Booth is on the radical fringe; to those who favor home birth and want to establish more freestanding birth centers, Booth is conservative. To the multitudes who are coming there from all sections of Philadelphia and environs to have their babies, Booth is a godsend.

As Kitty Ernst of MCA and Mabel Forde of Booth describe it, establishing Booth was an attempt to create a place "where not only can parents have power in making decisions that affect them, but providers can look at what is essential for the safety of mother and baby and what is desired to make childbirth a meaningful, confidence-building experience for parents" ("Maternity Care: An Attempt at an Alternative," *Nursing Clinics of North America,* June, 1975).

Booth is a four-floor residential hospital, run by the Salvation Army until 1971 for unwed mothers. Decline in demand for those services coincided with the development in Philadelphia and elsewhere of ideas favoring alternative maternity care. With the consulting help of MCA's Kitty Ernst and the direction of Dr. John Franklin of Jefferson University Hospital, this family-centered, parent-responsive, single-class, nurse-midwife-oriented facility was launched.

The Booth staff emphasizes the idea of the obstetrical team. There are nine full-time nurse-midwives, several part-time interns or refresher nurse-midwives, three obstetricians, and many nurses. Pediatricians from Jefferson University Hospital rotate in being available in case of infant distress.

Approximately 35 resident clients, mostly teenagers, receive the same prenatal care as the large and ever-growing group of couples and other singles who are coming to use Booth's program.

Maternity centers usually insist on a single class of care. At Booth the cost is $1750 ($1200 for hospital stay, $550 for doctors' fees) for everyone, excluding special tests or procedures. About 40% of Booth users have Medical Assistance coverage, 30% have Blue Cross or other insurance, and 30% self-pay.

The two delivery rooms are basically hospital operating rooms. The labor rooms can accommodate two women at a time. Booth Maternity Center is equipped like a hospital—it is a hospital—so there are fetal heart monitors (two of them) which get used in any labor where there is distress or concern and to check briefly on normal labors. Caesarean sections are of course performed.

As you might expect, the heart of the Booth situation is nurse-midwifery, and this is one major difference between it and standard hospital obstetric units. Prenatal care is in the nurse-midwives' capable hands, except for the two visits (minimum) a client will have with the obstetrician, one early in pregnancy and one toward the end. Prenatal visits are scheduled for evenings and weekends as well as weekday time so that working men and women can find a time to attend together. Midwives do a lot of educating and counseling in these visits—nutrition, physiology, newborn care, anything the family wants to talk about.

The midwives who teach the prenatal classes are the same women who attend a laboring woman (or a couple) during the whole childbirth experience. At Booth, the midwives catch the babies, unless the client prefers to have the obstetrician do it, or unless there is a complication like multiple birth or breech presentations.

Booth midwives will be running a newly planned facility within the Center as soon as it is completed. A homelike maternity care program, with liberal family orientation, will be located in a few separate rooms (like an apartment) in the same building as the hospital itself.

At Booth, preparation for childbirth is considered an essential part of care. (Compare this to the outright hostility that some doctors in private practice often reveal when patients discuss wanting to go to childbirth education classes!) ''Parents [at Booth] unable to attend any classes, or resistant to structured class instruction, are taught basic relaxation and breathing techniques during prenatal examinations, and are given intensive support and on-the-spot instruction in labor," write Ernst and Forde. Most Booth mothers are open to the idea of preparation. Booth is known as a "natural childbirth" facility, but there is considerable variation, just the same, in the level of preparation. No one is pushed into any one kind of approach to labor.

An outstanding feature of the Booth experience is the notion of the contract which the staff and the client develop as their mode of interaction. The client's chart is open and available. Needs, wishes, and fears, as well as medical information, are recorded on the chart, and the shared concern is simple: as Dr. Franklin expressed it, people should have the childbirth experience they want, within the guidelines of safe medical practice.

What is important are your feelings about your delivery experience, suggests Dr. Franklin. At Booth, the top-of-the-pyramid position for the doctor is underplayed. He or she doesn't *direct* the experience. The intent is to oversee conscious, active, mother-controlled birth. Toward the end of labor the doctor might step into the delivery room to see how things are going and then stand by the door for a while once the baby has started down the birth canal. Available with tools and knowledge, the doctor assumes the part of a backup person and advisor.

This spring I was meeting regularly with Dr. Franklin to chat about childbirth and ask medical and theoretical questions related to the writing of this book. One day, in the midst of one such conversation in his office at Booth, the phone buzzed, Dr. Franklin answered it, disappeared into the bathroom, emerged wearing OR clothes, and walked out the door. The other folks in the office and I talked among ourselves until Dr. Franklin reappeared barely half an hour later. "Did you just deliver a baby?" I asked, surprised. "No," he said, "Roslyn [one of the midwives] did, or rather the mother did, and Roslyn helped."

I attended a six-session prenatal class at Booth, taught by Carol Paruch, CNM, from Nova Scotia. It was a warm, pleasant, and educational experience. We saw films, practiced breathing and relaxation exercises, watched Carol describe the opening of the cervix using a knitted model of a uterus, and waited eagerly for the class parents to start delivering.

One of Carol's lessons impressed me particularly. In rehearsing for the contractions of labor, husbands (or other support persons) would exert a painful, pinching pressure on the ankle or knee of the pregnant woman, who would then practice breathing techniques to keep calm and help her cope with the discomfort. One evening Carol told the class to reverse roles. The men had a chance to act out the laboring woman's role while the women were able to practice the kind of eye contact and close connecting presence that they were beginning to realize they would need. Understanding the principle of substitution, of empathy, is a vital part of being a good labor-support person. Their subsequent experiences confirmed for many of these husbands just how thoroughly useful they could be during the birth process.

A first-time father, Jack, came back to the last session of our class and told his story of the birth of his child early that morning. As he spoke, his elation made him keep tripping over his words; he kept referring to "me" when he meant "her," his wife, Janet.

His first comment: "The people here are phenomenal, all the midwives and doctors are phenomenal, they keep you on top, they tell you it's ideal. For us," Jack said, "there were complications, our plans had to change, had to shift. Even then they just kept it going, right along."

Janet's cervix was tight and the baby was in posterior position. No real progress occurred over several hours after her water broke; Pitocin was administered. Three hours later, the contractions were strong, unrelenting in the way that drug-induced contractions often are. This was when Jack understood what Carol had regularly cautioned—that any given labor is not going to be like a textbook. Each labor has its own character.

Janet had the shakes; she was given a small dose of tranquilizer for relaxation. It was very difficult for her to get on top of these contractions. As labor progressed into transition, the internal lead from the fetal heart monitor was introduced. Janet was in considerable back pain (a usual posterior-labor complaint). Jack described vividly the work he did, with all his strength, on massaging her back. Janet told me later that she could never have done it without him.

The labor continued, the pushing began, the head crowned, the cord, around the neck, was quickly cut, and Alexandra came into the world.

"It's scary at times," Jack said. "We really needed to be together, with the midwife too, eye contact, and encouragement, and touching. We knew what to expect with the Pitocin, and that made it so much easier."

"Listen to what the midwives say!" he exhorted the class. Jack had taken Booth's labor guide sheet right through labor with him, and used it when coaching Janet's breathing.

"If your labor is not quite normal, like ours, the midwives will tell you what to do and you should do what they say, they have concern for how you feel and for what you think you are capable of. Nothing was routine. This place is phenomenal!"

Story: Margaret and John

I met Margaret and John for the first time when they arrived at Booth midway during labor one hot Sunday in July. That day I had been following Ruth Wilf, CNM, on her rounds.

It was a busy day. Ruth had spent the morning with a couple enduring miscarriage. She had gone from there to visit a young woman whose just-born daughter would be adopted soon, helping her to understand some of the feelings accompanying this experience. A delightful young couple asked Ruth about visitor policy, eager to share their 12-hour-old daughter with family and friends. I sat in on a talk Ruth was having with a primaparous couple in their early thirties whose anxiety about nursing was mounting with the approach of their return home—how could they best manage their well-meaning but discouraging relatives who had already advised the mother that her attempt to breastfeed would surely be unsuccessful? Ruth had some good supportive advice for them.

Then, around 1:30 in the afternoon, Margaret and John came in. Margaret is a large woman, in her late twenties; John is about the same age. They were concentrating hard and were nervous. Margaret had been thinking for a day or so that she was in labor; this time it seemed to be for real. She was clearly uncomfortable. In the examining room she found she was 6 to 7 cm dilated, good news. Her labor was well underway.

Margaret settled in a double labor room, glad to be out of the 96-degree heat, relieved to be in true labor at last. John settled down beside her, and Ruth introduced me to them. In this way Margaret and John acquired me as an extra fixture at their birthing just a few hours before young Jon was born; it was extra generous of them to have me there.

Ruth, cheerful and chatty, remarked at how relaxed Margaret was becoming now that she had settled in the labor bed, and Margaret smiled a genuine smile of relief. Ruth set about filling out the stack of papers, charts, and labels that must accompany every labor.

As part of her unobtrusive (but never secret) checking, the midwife keeps track of the baby's heartbeat. For a change from the stethoscope, Ruth applied some jelly to Margaret's abdomen, pressed the disk of the fetal heart monitor against Margaret's abdomen, and then engaged the ''on'' button of the stereo-like monitoring machine. Immediately, we were all hearing the loud, quick thump of the heart of Margaret and John's unborn baby. The monitor works by picking up sonar (sound) waves sent across water and transmitted back as a signal;

simultaneously a red light lights up with each heartbeat. Further, on the fhm a digital number flickers, changing numerals each second—147, 135, 136—numbering the per-minute beats based on each second's reading. Altogether, this use of the fetal heart monitor provided reassuring witness to the strength of the baby, and we all laughed and relaxed and enjoyed it. Then Ruth switched on the "record" button, and a pen drew a wavy line across graph paper at the level of 140, 122, 99, 111, and so forth. Another, yet different, reading of the same good news.

This baby was not in distress; there was no need to do extensive monitoring. Ruth removed the disk, wiped the jelly off, and said that John and Margaret could have the tracing for a souvenir if they would like.

At this point, Margaret's contractions were about 4 minutes apart. An internal exam revealed that in the past hour or two she had opened up only one more centimeter, that is, to 7 or 8 cm. It was here that Ruth suggested to walk to stimulate the labor. Somewhat reluctantly, Margaret agreed and with John's help slowly got herself out of the bed.

I walked with them down the hall, stopping for a contraction or two, past the nursery where one or two babies were sleeping. They spoke of their ten-year-old son, his hope for a brother. For that first birth, Maragret said, John hadn't been with her; this time he was, and she said she really preferred childbirth the companionable way.

There was a stop at the bathroom. Margaret had the fear that I think many laboring women have—that what will come out in the toilet is the baby. There are stories of this happening; but mostly the fear arises from sensorial confusions associated with the pushing or easing out of anything from the pelvis.

The midwives at Booth and at similar maternity facilities work in shifts, overlapping and usually extended. Generally shifts range from 7 to 3, 8 to 4, 11 to 7, and so forth. The change of midwife during a woman's labor may or may not upset her.

It was 3:30 now, past time for a shift change. I was sorry to see Ruth go and Ruth was sorry to go and perhaps Margaret would have been more comfortable if Ruth had stayed for continuity. Ruth said she really doesn't like to leave in the middle of a labor; if Margaret had got as far as the pushing stage, she would have remained for a while longer. After a final, quick internal examination, Ruth turned the labor attendance over to Anna. Ellen, an apprentice midwife who had just finished midwifery training in England after a nurse's training here, was also present carefully noticing everything Anna did.

The level of control Margaret had been able to exercise over the contractions at 7 cm dilatation was insufficient toward the end of first-stage labor. Transition really hit Margaret. She and John had not gone to childbirth preparation class. Margaret felt great pain, disbelief, and disorientation. She became increasingly unhappy, asked for relief, and spoke of her suffering with surprise, frustration, and even anger. The midwives gently reminded her to keep breathing with a "hout" and to keep her eyes open, looking at her husband. But the kind of teamwork which builds up over those practice sessions at childbirth preparation class can't usually be constructed on the spot for the couple who has not prepared. John was, I think, feeling powerless to help his wife in her pain and unhappiness. I reminded her of breathing when I could; the midwives assured her from time to time that the end was in sight. I was aware more than ever of the importance of the coach's role and the value to the laboring woman of having a trained companion.

After several cries for help from Margaret, Anna, who was being the midwife in charge, decided in consultation with the doctor on hand the give a very small I.V. dose of Demerol to help Margaret relax between contractions. That is precisely what the Demerol did. Although Margaret reported no appreciable diminishing of pain, she was able to doze off between contractions. This very effect has been the object of criticism from women who have been given Demerol—you are so groggy, they say, that you lose the ability to get on top of each or any contraction. Margaret's undiminished call for relief resulted in a second dose of Demerol, although the midwives were visibly reluctant to administer this. Their decision to do so was based most of all on Margaret's own wish to further reduce her discomfort.

To be sure, not everyone who gives birth at Booth (or any facility, for that matter) holds not being medicated as a strict value. Indeed, the estimates I received about medication at Booth, in whatever quantity, are in the 80% range. For Margaret, the Demerol made her feel less frantic and quieter. The two doses, 12.5 cc each, totaled about one third of that which most hospitals routinely give; so in a comparative sense Margaret's was yet a "small" dose.

Margaret like most laboring women, seemed to find the pushing a relief after the trials of late first-stage labor. The delivery room crew coached her efforts. With each contraction she got two, and sometimes three, strong pushes in. And she wasn't holding back on making sounds, either, something many women have a problem with. Like a driver struggling to push her car out of a deep rut, or a karate student learning to focus all muscle tension and mind concentration at a moment, Margaret knew instinctively to let the noise emerge, from the abdomen—to summon and gather together the large effort of her whole person. Obstetrician Joni Magee (of Booth), in an article called "Labor: What the Doctor Learns as a Patient" (*The Female Patient,*

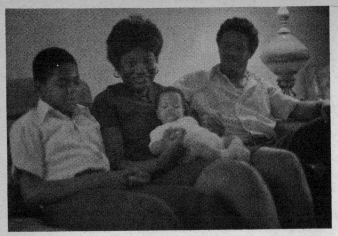

Margaret and John and Landon and Jon.

*1:*11), writes about her own labor and suggests to her colleagues that they encourage women to moan and groan, that to let the grunts and gurgles come out can be of help. It was for Margaret. She worked hard and well, looking regularly to her husband for the hand-holding and reassurance he was glad to give her.

The baby inched its way down the birth canal. In between second-stage contractions most women rest. A woman who has had Demerol, as we have noted, dozes off; this was Margaret's state. Her baby was nearing the end of its descent. An injection of local anesthetic was then given for an episiotomy. There was a snip of the scissors and, in a moment, the boy himself came sliding out, 5:11 P.M., lovely and lively, Jon.

I can't say for sure which midwife caught Jon. I was watching open-mouthed as the baby's head emerged.

No traction was used on the cord. After the placenta was out, there flowed a steady stream of bright red blood. Hemorrhage was the one thought on my mind, and I could see some concern among the midwives and the obstetrical nurse. The bleeding, however, soon stopped.

Margaret was surprised when they said she could hold her baby. She did, there on the table, and he sucked, and that mother looked very pleased indeed. Yet as Margaret lay there she told Anna she was changing her mind, that she did not think she would breastfeed after all. I didn't want to interfere, but I did anyway, and urged her to talk the next day with Ruth or any of the midwives before making a decision for sure.

And there was John grinning, proud, quiet. He made the acquaint-

ance of his new son, being warmed by lights, and he shook hands with
the obstetrician who had been standing by in the doorway just in case.

COMPARATIVE COSTS AND INSURANCE

Generally, for services operated largely by Certified Nurse-Midwives,
fees are significantly lower than the fees for a private physician/hos-
pital arrangement. Table I gives estimates, for the most part, for some
selected facilities. Prices have a way of changing fast, so use this only
as a guide, not as gospel.

TABLE I Cost According to Facility

Facility or Type of Facility	Cost in $	What Is Included
Urban high-risk center (MCA estimate)	700	Obstetrician's fee
	1300	Hospital stay
	30	Each prenatal visit
Roosevelt Hospital in New York, midwife-staffed service	1179	Everything (excluding abnormal problems): prenatal labor and delivery, 2-day hospital stay
MCA, New York Childbearing Center	885	Everything, including postpartum care
Midwife-staffed home delivery service (MCA, Maryland)	500	Everything, including postpartum care
High-risk teaching hospital, clinic maternity care	700	3-day stay, clinic visits, labor and delivery
Same high-risk teaching hospital, private care	500	Obstetrician's fee
	850	Hospital stay
	1800	Same as above, but with Caesarean
Booth Maternity Center	1750	Everything, including postpartum; 4-day stay

The exact terms of coverage by Medical Assistance, Medicare, Medi-caid, and health insurance policies are of course, essential for your figuring.

From insurance companies, basically three different kinds of options are available for maternity coverage.

(1) Companies that only give complications coverage unless you pay specifically for maternity coverage. One policy for pregnancy benefits *for complications only* stipulates the following: Benefits are provided for charges in connection with certain complications of pregnancy of any female covered under this Major Medical Plan, whether the Maternity Benefit option is selected or not. These eligible charges are—

    (a) Services and supplies, required during hospital confinement, solely for treatment of pernicious vomiting of pregnancy or toxemia with convulsions.

    (b) The following surgical services and related services and supplies required after surgery: Caesarean section after the sixth month of pregnancy, intra-abdominal surgery after pregnancy terminates, operation for extra-uterine pregnancy.

The pregnancy must begin while the female is covered under the plan.

(2) If you pay specifically for maternity coverage, according to the same company as (1) above, the following maternity benefits are included: When a female insured or a dependent female spouse is eligible, benefits are payable—

    (a) Up to the available level of protection you select for eligible charges for a normal delivery;

    (b) One and a half times this level for charges for Caesarean section or extra-uterine pregnancy;

    (c) One half this level for charges for an abortion or miscarriage.

This plan covers pregnancies which begin when the person has been covered for at least 30 days prior thereto. Also, benefits are not afforded unless the hospitalization occurs and the obstetrical procedure is performed while she is covered.

(3) Companies like Blue Cross provide maternity benefits when you buy their package. With this arrangement, pregnancy benefits are available to applicant subscriber or spouse after eight months' enrollment under a family contract. One such policy stipulates the following coverage:

    (a) Full semi-private benefits for mother and child for up to six days during each pregnancy.

    (b) Delivery room and nursery care included.

    (c) Newborn child is entitled to full service benefits up to 50 to 120 days, including:

       —nursery care in the treatment for illness;

—congenital defects;
—prematurity;
—postmaturity;
—circumcision.

(d) Full semi-private benefits for up to ten days for Caesarean birth, miscarriage or premature termination of pregnancy not resulting in childbirth. Fifty to 120 days are available for an ectopic pregnancy.

TABLE II EXPENSES OF THE THREE COUPLES

People	Cost in $	What Was Included
Loretta and Zak	500	Obstetrician's fee, $90 covered by Blue Shield
	1000	Hospital costs, 5-day stay, almost all covered by Blue Cross
Sue and Jonah	400	Obstetrician's and midwife's fee (usually 450, but Sue and Jonah signed up late in Sue's pregnancy); includes prenatal care
Margaret and John	1200	Booth standard fee (in 1976)

6

Childbirth Education Resources

A primary source of information about childbirth is mothers, mothers and fathers, neighbors and friends and relatives, people who will share with you experiences they have had. These offerings can be uniquely valuable. You should be cautioned, however, against signing up for one kind of childbirth experience—a particular doctor, a method of preparation—simply on the basis that the experience so well suited someone you know.

Perhaps the most valuable contribution that your recently-delivered friends will have to offer is specific leads for you to follow. Check these out for how they feel to *you*.

Remember, too, that you are in every way allowed to change your mind and take your obstetrical business elsewhere if you are uncomfortable with your arrangements.

Change, after all, is the order of the day in maternal care, thanks largely to the work of parent/professional organizations such as the ones described in this chapter. Your friend Kate's episiotomy at the local hospital six or seven years ago may well have been unnecessary, unquestioned, "routine." Today, at the critical moment in your delivery—same obstetrician and same hospital—you just might be part of the "team" deciding that you don't need that quite often elective procedure.

Moreover, because of the demands and the work of parents and professionals along with them, there are simply more choices available every year. Maternity centers and home birth are in their early years as organized phenomena with some medical approval and backup; neither was really anywhere to be seen in 1970.

No matter where you deliver, no matter whose hands catch the baby, the more you know, the better prepared you are, the better it will go for you. Education and preparation are the first tasks of a careful pregnancy.

Education for childbirth has empirical advantages. Doris Haire, in *The Cultural Warping of Childbirth* refers to research carried out by Dr. Murray Enkin (a director of ICEA) in the Toronto area, demonstrating that ". . . mothers who were prepared for the possibility of effectively participating in the birth process tended to experience significantly shorter labors, to require less medication and less obstetrical intervention and to remember the experience of birth more favorably than did those mothers who were motivated to ask to be prepared to cope with childbirth but could not be accommodated in classes.''

Comparatively speaking, however, we still in this culture have some distance to go in making sure that all childbearing couples have solid access to childbirth education.

The Bibliography (Chapter 8) includes many books that are good resources in this effort. This chapter examines resources of other kinds: classes, organizations, and the media, with a word about some enlightening childbirth resources for children.

CHILDBIRTH EDUCATION CLASSES

In the 1830s and 1840s, when lay healers were losing business to the rising profession of medicine, there arose the Popular Health Movement described by Ehrenreich and English in their excellent pamphlet *Witches, Midwives and Nurses.* Women, it seems, were the backbone of the movement. Self-help anatomy and hygiene courses sprang up; some elements of the movement were even discussing birth control. The Popular Health Movement was linked with the beginnings of the organized movement for women's rights, and joined with the working-class rejection of the elitism of medicine. There was much feeling in the Popular Health Movement that the practice of medicine was more appropriate to women than to men.

In our time, childbirth education as a movement, if not directly political, resembles in some ways the energy of that early, nearly forgotten effort, representing as it does the feelings and needs of people often up against the policies of established medicine, and dedicated as it is to basic information and self-help.

Barbara Brennan, Certified Nurse-Midwife at New York City's Roosevelt Hospital, estimates that approximately 50% of pregnant women in America today attend preparation classes. I have heard this same estimate from some other childbirth educators. In the oft-hailed Dutch system, special classes are sought less often than one would guess from their legendary good obstetrical outcomes. Since prenatal care among the Dutch people is usually in the hands of the midwives, education for birth occurs naturally as part of their prenatal care.

The French have a sensible attitude toward encouraging prenatal preparation. According to Aidan Macfarlane, M.D., in the epilogue

to *The Psychology of Childbirth*, the French government gives
" . . . benefits to parents of between $1200 and $1800 if they attend
an antenatal clinic and bring the child for regular checkups over the
first year of his life . . . a far sighted investment in economic terms,
for high attendance at the clinics has reduced the incidence of death
and handicap, and the government has to spend less on the provision
of special homes and facilities."

In parts of Canada, on the other hand, the acceptance by doctors of
prepared childbirth has been a less regulated, more gradual process.
Betsy in rural Ontario, a journalist, anthropologist, and mother,
pointed out that doctors in her area responded favorably to the idea of
prepared childbirth when a local newspaper did a survey on attitudes:
" . . . inquiries of women in the maternity section of the hospital I
went to, however, suggested that many doctors do not do anything to
ensure that their patients receive training prior to labor or to ensure
that 'trained' parents do not receive drugs." Evidently it is one thing
to vote yes on a media survey and quite another to begin to accept
patients' questions and requests for special arrangement—and yet
another to actively encourage parent education and responsibility.
Betsy noted that although it had required no special arranging for her
and Tom to be together for the birth of their child, she was the only
one of seven women in labor at the time who had a companion along
with her.

In selecting a childbirth class from the mainstream of our North
American culture, you have two general kinds to consider: hospital
and independent.

American hospitals are relative newcomers in the field of childbirth
preparation courses. One early example is Flower-Fifth Avenue Hospital in New York which, though now defunct, offered its own
childbirth education starting in the 1960s. In less populated areas,
hospital classes have slowly been developing more recently. The
gradual recognition by physicians of the usefulness of such classes
has been a factor in their growth.

If you are planning for a hospital birth, the hospital where you will
be delivering may have its own series of classes. These usually meet
once a week for six or seven weeks.

Along with initiating you into the routines and specifics of that
particular hospital (which may include a heavier emphasis than you
would want on the need for drugs) such a series of classes is more and
more likely nowadays to have a curriculum oriented toward the
approaches of Dick-Read and Lamaze. Basic physiological information is given. There is usually some teaching of breathing techniques
for labor, relaxation exercises, and muscle-limbering exercises. Medications and procedures are described. Postpartum care, pediatric

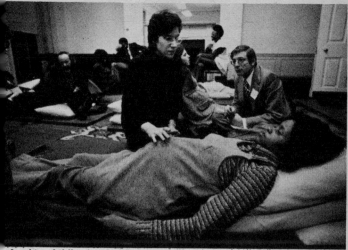

In this childbirth education class the instructor is explaining the usefulness of relaxation during first-stage labor.

needs, and perhaps breastfeeding are also considered. Most hospitals now accept the father as a legitimate member of the childbearing unit and welcome his class participation.

The final class of most hospital orientation courses is the hospital tour. This would be a good class to go to even if you have chosen a basic preparation class outside the hospital where you plan to deliver. You can spare yourself the possible anxiety of trying to settle down in labor in an unfamiliar setting if you have attended this tour and had your questions answered in advance.

Independent classes are the other usual source of childbirth education. Though they educate hospital-users about hospital routine, and though they are often more critical of medical intervention than a hospital course, independently taught classes have the disadvantage of not being able to prepare parents for the routines of a specific facility. So, in addition to attending such a class, you will have to inquire further and make your own contacts with the obstetrician and pediatrician at the hospital.

Apart from personal advice from friends, there are two ways to locate non-hospital classes: contact an organization such as the ones listed in this chapter, or consult the Yellow Pages. My city's Yellow Pages has an index heading ''Childbirth Education Preparation,'' followed by a cross-reference: ''See Social Service Organizations.''

The listings under "Social Service Organizations" fill one-and-a-half four-column pages; alphabetically under "Childbirth" is the entry for CEA and the entry for Lamaze, with local addresses and phone numbers.

Most childbirth education courses cost money, especially if they are independent of hospitals. The usual range is from $30 to $50 for a six-class series. Preparation offered at facilities which emphasize continuity of care and have nurse-midwives on staff usually include prenatal classes in their overall cost of services.

When you go looking for a class, you will do well to have in mind certain questions and standards. *Our Bodies, Ourselves* suggests a list of criteria, as does Valmai Elkins, the Montreal-based educator whose book *The Rights of the Pregnant Parent* has a considerable amount of useful consumer information. Following is a summary of the points made by both—criteria for choosing a childbirth education class:

(1) *Size*. Fewer than 10 couples is recommended; small classes encourage discussion.

(2) *Labor support*. Make sure the class encourages fathers or friends to participate, to be trained along with you as your coach.

(3) *Content*. Check that the course includes information on important topics, including nutrition, postpartum adjustment, psychological issues, breastfeeding. Be sure that sufficient time is given to rehearsal of breathing, exercises, and relaxation.

(4) *Duration*. Six weeks is minimal, seven or eight recommended.

(5) *Sponsor*. Find out as much as you can about the organization sponsoring or offering the classes, about the instructor and her/his references and her/his background. You may also want to get a feel for how strongly that person supports various concerns of prepared childbirth, such as avoidance of unnecessary medication.

If you can't get to a class, there are childbirth preparations available in book and recorded forms that would generally be sufficient. Books like Erna Wright's *The New Childbirth* and Dick-Read's *The Practice of Natural Childbirth* are compact childbirth education courses in themselves. Consult the Bibliography of this book for others. As mentioned under the story of Loretta and Zak in Chapter 5, a noted Lamaze instructor in the Philadelphia area has made a recording of her teachings. One couple told me they found the recordings even more helpful than the class itself for sustaining practicing and encouragement. ASPO (see under "Organizations," below) would be the source for such a recording.

What parents learn in class helps determine their way of involving themselves in the birth process when the time comes. When the preparation and the delivery are in the same hands, parents are spared the jarring experience that comes when expectations of labor and the reality of labor are dramatically different.

With these considerations in mind, here is a selection of the many energetic, committed, people-oriented groups who will further prepare and educate you.

ORGANIZATIONS

It is characteristic of childbirth associations that parents and professionals together found them and run them: ICEA, ASPO, ACHI, and NAPSAC all function in this dynamic way.

The following organizations are our sources of information about classes, educational materials, and much else. Further, they are agents of change in obstetrics in our society. Through their efforts, our voices as consumers can be joined. I include first those groups which are international and national, then selected regional/local groups. (For additional information about the groups listed below, consult the Index to this book.)

International Childbirth Education Association (ICEA, or CEA)
P.O. Box 20852
Milwaukee, Wisconsin 53220

ICEA Supplies Center
P.O. Box 70258
Seattle, Washington 98107

The International Childbirth Education Association, founded in 1960, is the most inclusive and the most widely known of the childbirth associations and groups. Its watchword is "Freedom of Choice Through Knowledge of Alternatives," and it announces that its primary aim is Family Centered Maternity Care.

The primary route to knowledge of alternative is the CEA prenatal course for parents. This course is offered in communities all over North America; looking in the telephone directory is one way to find the address and phone number of a local CEA group; writing to the main address, given above, is another.

CEA is really a federation of groups. The services it performs are numerous. CEA coordinates the activities of Nursing Mothers groups; has committees working on various newsletters, journals, and directories; runs the Supplies Center in Seattle, which puts out current booklists (free), and carries the best basic books; trains instructors;

has committees on father participation, pediatric care, aspects of parenting. CEA issues reports of local events, regional conferences, and national news.

Information about childbirth audio-visual materials can be obtained through the Supplies Center; they have available a *Directory of Films and Records*. A recording called "Practice for Childbirth," by Elisabeth Bing and Ferris Urbanowski, 1973, is available for $1.95.

An important facet of CEA work from the beginning has been its focus on consumer input to change policies in hospitals. Careful referral based on up-to-date documenting of parent experiences at local hospitals is part of the education CEA parents receive.

The list of educators, doctors, midwives, and physical therapists from all corners of the obstetric community who have at some point worked with CEA reads like a Who's Who in Childbirth: Elisabeth Bing, Roberto Caldeyro-Barcia, T. Berry Brazelton, Sheila Kitzinger, Marshall Klaus, Ruth Watson Lubic, Ashley Montagu, Niles Newton, Pierre Vellay, Murray Enkin, Doris Haire, Lester Hazell, John Franklin, Virginia Apgar, Ruth Wilf.

Maternity Center Association (MCA)
48 East 92nd Street
New York, New York 10028

In this country Maternity Center Association of New York, founded in 1918, has been the pioneer in promoting the cause of childbirth education and family-oriented, medically safe maternity care. Its work is described in Chapter 5 under the section "The Idea of the Maternity Center."

The publications (See Bibliography), films, and teaching aids of MCA represent one valuable aspect of its commitment to childbirth education. In addition, many of the new maternity centers all over the country look to MCA for consultation and informal coordination of information to be shared.

American Society for Psychoprophylaxis in Obstetrics (ASPO)
1411 K Street, NW
Washington, D.C. 20005

This is the official Lamaze organization, whose purpose is to spread knowledge of the Lamaze method (psychoprophylaxis) and direct the training of teachers of the method. Information about centers of Lamaze preparation throughout the country and Canada can be obtained from ASPO.

The Society was founded in 1960 through the concerted efforts of Elisabeth Bing, the well-known Lamaze teacher and writer, and

Marjorie Karmel, an American woman who had her first child in Paris with Dr. Lamaze, and soon after wrote *Thank You, Dr. Lamaze*.

La Leche League International (LLLI)
9616 Minneapolis Avenue
Franklin Park, Illinois 60131

There are over 2600 LLLI groups in the United States and other countries. Founded in 1957, the organization is dedicated, like the title of their classic work on the subject, to *The Womanly Art of Breastfeeding*.

The most important work of the League concerns the active support and education of nursing mothers by the method of personal contact: there is a practical four-meeting series, and networks of contact among mothers. La Leche (pronounced lay-chay) is the Spanish word for *milk*. LLLI also issues a news publication (available through subscription), operates a free book-lending service, and has a film called "Talking About Breastfeeding," which groups use in introducing the League's work.

National Association of Parents and Professionals
for Safe Alternatives in Childbirth (NAPSAC)
P.O. Box 267
Marble Hill, Missouri 63674

NAPSAC Childbirth Research Institute
P.O. Box 129
Cottage Grove, Wisconsin 53527

The cover photo (by Suzanne Arms) of the 1976 NAPSAC book *Safe Alternatives in Childbirth* is the image of this group's concern—a just-born baby held in a bath, looking up at us: here is a new person, in our hands.

NAPSAC is the group to consult for writing and research about family-centered, nonroutine obstetrics. Responsible medical knowledge and a strong commitment to family values in childbearing distinguish this organization. It publishes a quarterly newsletter and books on alternatives in childbirth, and also has film listings.

Dr. Lewis Mehl is the Director of the Research Institute of NAPSAC: its board of consultants includes Doris Haire, Lester Hazell, Nancy Mills, Dr. Gregory White, and Ruth Wilf, CNM, among others.

Another distinguishing feature of NAPSAC is its membership, drawn from parents, medical professionals, and childbirth educators. The goals of this productive, diverse group are to promote education about natural childbirth; to facilitate communication and cooperation among parents, medical professionals, and childbirth educators; to educate and aid in the creation of family-centered maternity care in hospitals; to help establish maternity and childbearing centers; to help establish safe home birth programs; and to provide educational opportunities to parents and parents-to-be "that will enable them to assume more personal responsibility for Pregnancy, Childbirth, Infant Care, and Child Rearing."

The 1977 NAPSAC book, like the 1976 one, is the collected proceedings of NAPSAC's annual meeting; it is a two volume resource, entitled *21st-Century Obstetrics Now*.

Association for Childbirth at Home, International (ACHI)
16705 Monte Cristo *or* Box 1219
Cerritos, California 90701

This organization, growing rapidly, was founded in 1972 in Boston by Tonya Brooks, who is still its president. The group (until 1977 known as Association for Childbirth at Home, ACAH) is dedicated to support of, encouragement of, and education for childbirth at home. Research on all aspects of home birth is conducted and analyzed by ACHI; leader-training is also conducted. Through its more than 100 local groups here and in Canada, ACHI offers a six-session, $40 course open to prospective parents and to professionals interested in home birth; the course combines the standard information of prenatal classes with special information and preparation regarding birth at home.

ACHI issues "Birth Notes," an informative newsletter with articles of practical concern. The organization maintains regional headquarters, at least one of which operates a mail-order bookstore with well-selected titles. Write to: ACAH Bookstore, c/o John & Sue Crockett, 69 Moseman Avenue, Katonah, New York, 10536.

On the Board of Advisors of ACHI: Dr. Tom Brewer, Sheila Kitzinger, David and Lee Stewart of NAPSAC, Ruth Wilf, CNM, Ashley Montagu, Doris Haire.

American Academy of Husband-Coached Childbirth (AAHCC)
P.O. Box 5224
Sherman Oaks, California

This organization came to being with the popularity of Dr. Robert A. Bradley's book *Husband-Coached Childbirth*. Its aim is to teach a technique of natural childbirth that emphasizes the active, emotional and coaching participation of the father; Bradley also teaches muscle relaxation and mental distraction techniques for the woman during active labor. The organization trains instructors in the Bradley method; AAHCC instructors now teach in Mexico and Australia as well as in the United States and Canada.

AAHCC has films on nutrition and childbirth that are available for sale or rent. Details on teacher-training, workshops, lectures, and films are all handled at the above address.

Planned Parenthood Federation of America, Inc.
515 Madison Avenue
New York, New York 10022

This large organization has services throughout the country, offering clinic care, free libraries, extensive referrals. From the national headquarters come publications and research in family planning, pregnancy, childbirth, gynecology, and related areas.

National Foundation/March of Dimes
P.O. Box 2000
White Plains, New York 10602

The March of Dimes has been dedicated to services regarding birth defects for many decades. They publish bulletins and pamphlets on the Rh factor, rubella (German measles), drugs, birth defects, etc., and they are a source for filmstrips. The March of Dimes directs people to genetic counseling services and to medical/social services for victims of birth defects.

The late Virginia Apgar, M.D., author of *Is My Baby All Right?*, served as Vice President for Medical Affairs of the March of Dimes.

Society for the Protection of the Unborn through Nutrition (SPUN)
17 North Wabash, Suite 603
Chicago, Illinois 60602

Dr. Tom Brewer is the guiding light of this organization. Its concerns have been summarized by *Mothering* magazine: ''SPUN recognizes that the universal application of scientific prenatal care, which includes nutrition education, will markedly reduce the incidence of birth tragedies by tens of thousands. If we would begin to emphasize preventive medicines as much as we do symptomatic medicine and crisis medicine, much of the anguish experienced by families of brain damaged children as well as the devastating social and economic toll of preventable maternal and infant disease, damage, and death could be avoided.''

The organization sponsors films and speakers, has produced a flyer ''Pregnant? and Want a Healthy Child?'' and puts out a biweekly newsletter and bibliographies of scientific studies.

American College of Home Obstetrics (ACHO)
664 North Michigan Avenue, Suite 600
Chicago, Illinois 60611

The American College of Home Obstetrics was founded, as stated
by NAPSAC, to "gather together those physicians who wish to
cooperate with families who choose to give birth in the home, the
natural and traditional place for birth throughout the world and the
ages." The physicians who are members are dedicated to learning
from and teaching to each other the "art of the safe supervision of
homebirths." ACHO seeks to foster the welfare of not only mother
and baby, but the whole family together. Dr. Gregory White, author
of *Emergency Childbirth,* is president.

Home Oriented Maternity Experience (HOME)
511 New York Avenue
Takoma Park, Washington, D.C. 20012

This group emphasizes the new responsibilities that parents are
taking on themselves in deciding to give birth at home, "reclaiming
their right to manage and maintain control over their labors, deliveries
and post-partum periods." Active participation of the father is
stressed by HOME. Centered around community meetings, the organization offers advice about how to do the best you can with hospital
birth; its newsletter, for instance, lists what to request from the
hospital, maintaining the same attitudes toward birth there as in the
home.

The manual put out by HOME is called *Home Oriented Maternity
Experience;* it is a paperback by Dorothy Fitzgerald, et al., and costs
$3.50. It is available from ICEA Supplies Center, at the address given
at the beginning of this section.

American Foundation for Maternal and Child Health, Inc.
30 Beekman Place
New York, New York 10022

This organization is concerned with public protection against the
hazards of drugs, procedures, interventions. The group offers
research findings and is a resource for proceedings of conferences on
topics of concern in maternity care.

Along with local chapters of national organizations like ICEA,
ASPO, LLLI, and ACHI, you may find some local organizations
which are devoted to childbirth education and community-minded
sharing of information and advice and resources. Some examples
follow.

In Boston: BACE, the Boston Association for Childbirth Education, with which Constance Bean, educator and author, has been involved; and Birth Day, a home birth group. In Montreal: MCEA, the Montreal Childbirth Education Association, which was started in 1972 by Valmai Elkins, the author of *The Rights of the Pregnant Parent*, and which has been very active in changing hospital policy in the Montreal area as well as educating the public in general by lectures and workshops. In Toronto: SACH, or Safe Alternative Childbirth at Home. Sources of information about these local groups would be the CEA group in the area, Planned Parenthood, any women's health clinic.

Center for Family Growth
555 Highland Avenue
Cotati, California 94928

The focus of the work of this local organization is spiritual, yogic, herbal. The most recent word I had from Jeannine O'Brien Medvin (who wrote the *Prenatal Yoga* manual I include in the Bibliography) announced the opening of a counseling-oriented Wholistic Prenatal Clinic and Midwifery Training Program as part of what they call the Birth and Death Center. Another present interest of the group is "natural" birth control.

C/SEC
c/o Pat Erickson
23 Cedar Street
Cambridge, Massachusetts 02140

Here is a local resource for information and support concerning Caesarean birth. C/SEC stands for Caesareans/Support, Education, and Concern.

There is now a movement in women's health—not surprising, since women consume significantly more health care than men. This movement has organizations and publications at national, regional, and local levels. Included here are those resources which serve at a national level.

National Women's Health Network
P.O. Box 24192
Washington, D.C. 20024

This national coordinating group, which appeared in 1976, is a health resource group, focusing on legislation, informing the public, organizing local community work on health care issues of women. It publishes "Network News."

The Women's Health Forum (Healthright)
175 Fifth Avenue
New York, New York 10010

This forum publishes *Healthright,* a newsletter of the women's health movement, and many pamphlets and flyers. The work of the Forum also includes courses and workshops on all aspects of women's health.

Feminist Women's Health Centers
112 Crenshaw Boulevard
Los Angeles, California 90005

Coordinators of women's health clinics all over the U.S., this group is the headquarters of a national network. Local clinics usually offer basic gynecology and are beginning to consider setting up maternity services. In Philadelphia, the Elizabeth Blackwell Health Center for Women offers full gynecological services, pregnancy tests, and counseling services; since mid-1977, plans have been under way to establish obstetrical care. Coordinating the clinic part of maternity care with the labor/delivery part, which would take place at a hospital nearby, is a challenge; this is the next step.

Boston Women's Health Book Collective, Inc.
Box 192
West Somerville, Massachusetts 02144

In the spring of 1969 this group of women planned a summer research project on women's health. From this came *Our Bodies, Ourselves,* now in its Second Edition, Completely Revised and Expanded, published in several European countries and Japan, hailed as a classic, a must, a milestone in women's health—easily the single most important book available on women's health.

The collective provides other health education work, a vigilant review of the media for information on all aspects of women's health. They have aided my own research with up-to-date clippings in maternity care news.

THE MEDIA

Films, television, magazines

Childbirth education films are usually distributed through such organizations as the ICEA.

The film of this sort which I have encountered most often is "The Story of Eric," in which an average pleasant-young-couple after slight complications successfully have their baby in a hospital with Lamaze method teachings and the cooperation of their very progressive obstetrician.

An unusual and excellent birth sequence occurs in the documentary film called "The Chicago Maternity Center Story," which I describe in Chapter 5. Kartemquin/Haymarket, 1901 West Wellington, Chicago, Illinois, made and distributes this film.

ACHI distributes some of its Super-8 films of home births. Their newsletter lists "Welcome to Our World," for instance, a 17-minute film, which sells for $75. Most films are for rent as well as for sale.

Drs. Klaus and Kennell at Case Western Reserve have collaborated, with others, on a film which we saw at the Booth Maternity Center prenatal class: called "The Amazing Newborn," it examines the complexity, responsiveness, and range of abilities that researchers are discovering in the newborn.

Another childbirth film which extends the content of childbirth education classes is called "Are You Ready for the Post-Partum Experience?" It carefully presents some of the difficulties in adjustment that all families can expect after the addition of a new baby.

"A Child Is Born" is a film of the Leboyer method in action that has been shown on Canadian Television. MCA or ICEA would be a source of information for this.

MCA, not surprisingly, came up with a prize-winning, basic education film in 1959: called "Generation to Generation," it is still shown widely today. MCA has also shown a videotape about midwives called "The Baby-Catchers."

A look at what appeared on national and local commercial and educational television during the nine months (yes) I have been working on this book reveals quite a variety of childbirth information coming over the airwaves into our living rooms. I saw a local (UHF channel) show in which a Bradley-trained physician and a Lamaze-oriented physician debated the relative merits of their styles. NBC-TV in February, 1977, aired a special called "Miracles in Childbirth," dramatically detailing some of the remarkable life-saving, high-risk procedures we now have, such as amniocentesis and sound-wave pictures of the fetus *in utero*. A local special news report examined delivery at a hospital in the area where nurse-midwives have been put on the staff.

ABC-TV locally presented a documentary of a New Jersey couple in their CEA preparation and hospital birth. This show, called "Johnny Victor's Birthday," represents some big changes in mass consciousness about birth. The father in the film is instructed by the obstetrician (who announces that his own job is to "stand by"), and it is the father who catches the baby. Considerable space is given to the CEA preparation of the couple. Though the actual birth sequence was obscured by drapes, on the whole the values of active participation by the father and of childbirth preparation classes were substantially supported in this presentation.

"Giving Birth," an hour-long documentary produced by Global Village in New York and shown on National Educational Television early in 1977, presented four births in their particulars, interspersing interviews with prominent figures in philosophy and obstetric practice today. The choices made by the four couples included one home birth, two hospital births, and one maternity center birth, covering the range of options facing today's expectant parents.

Frederick Leboyer, the compassionate and controversial French obstetrician, speaks on this videotape of the growth of his philosophy. Margaret Mead, in an interview, stresses the need for not removing the woman from active participation. Other experts from different areas of obstetrics give their views, and the births speak for themselves.

It is a remarkable program, richly informative, and full of great emotional moments.

"Having Babies," an ABC-TV movie written by Peggy Elliott, also follows four births. In this case, however, the format is fiction, not documentary. A shared Lamaze class is what brings together the four couples, with their different life situations and reasons for choosing Lamaze preparation: one an unmarried woman befriended by her widower neighbor; one a young couple choosing to give birth at home and struggling with the woman's father's disapproval of their lifestyle; one a widower father of three and his new wife who endure an emergency Caesarean resulting in stillbirth; and one a wealthy young lawyer and his unhappy wife, who comes to recognize her dissatisfaction with having given up her sports career. The last of these couples is the only one whose delivery is shown on film; it includes a (hasty) Leboyer bath.

In this presentation, facts about labor and the actual content of the Lamaze classes are subordinate to the dramatic material. But the show manages to be informative and further testifies to popular interest in and growing acceptance of the idea of preparation for childbirth.

A substantial book could be written about the coverage in popular media of issues in childbirth: how the incidence of magazine articles on midwives or midwifery began to grow in the late sixties and early seventies, and similarly with articles about "natural" childbirth.

In the June 28, 1977, issue of *Woman's Day* magazine, for instance, appeared an article by Fredelle Maynard called "Home Birth vs. Hospital Birth," in which the idea of home birth is given a full and positive treatment, with appropriate medical cautions and explanations. Such an article would not have appeared even five years ago, when home birth was a choice too radical and limited to make it newsworthy.

Magazines such as *Woman's Day, Redbook,* and *McCall's* regularly include articles on topics like childbirth, pregnancy, and childrearing. These summarize current findings on issues of concern and direct readers to organizations, books, and other resources. One of the best voices ever heard on any such topic (and on lots of others) was that of Margaret Mead, the American anthropologist who for more than forty years educated us about family life in many cultures. Dr. Mead wrote a regular column for *Redbook;* by chance at Planned Parenthood one day I picked up an old issue, and there was an article by Mead about single-parent families—basic, wise, penetrating.

Ms., a popular women's magazine which began in 1972, has published good criticism of books written for children about sexuality and reproduction. Its format offers the reader researched documentary articles on the one hand, and personal experience articles on the other. In the December, 1976, issue, there is a story by Barbara Katz Rothman, "In Which a Sensible Woman Persuades Her Doctor, Her Family, and Her Friends To Help Her Give Birth At Home." It is witty and well presented.

A few magazine pieces not from the "popular" media are worthy of note here.

"Labor: What the Doctor Learns as a Patient" is a valuable article, written by obstetrician Joni Magee (of Booth Maternity Center), in which she calls to the attention of doctors the feelings a laboring woman has. Her information is direct and concrete. Magee expresses her intention: "I should like to pass some of these ideas on to physicians who, because of inclination and/or anatomy, are limited to the medical view."

Her recommendations are simple enough, and if followed by obstetricians would, I am sure, reduce the fear and discomfort of many a laboring woman: pay attention to the mother; explain what you are doing; do internal exams just before a contraction instead of at the height of one; and so forth. She also recommends that the obstetrician encourage women in labor to scream out if they wish, when something painful is happening; Magee has found that this can help the woman feel better, and helps her feel that the doctor is on her side.

This article, brief though it is, has a special significance. Magee is in a minority position in her field (about 97% of obstetricians are men). Based on her own experience of labor, these simple, clear directions about how to make the bond of trust between patient and doctor more effective are a useful contribution; and who could refute her information?

The magazine in which this article appears is called *The Female Patient* (December, 1976), designed for health professionals who care primarily for women. (The advertisements for drugs in this magazine tell a tale of their own.)

A magazine called *Women & Health* has published its first issue, in which there is a good article on midwifery. This publication, which includes reviews of relevant books and films, is both scholarly and feminist.

There is one magazine devoted entirely to mothering, and that is its name: *Mothering: Sharings on Natural Motherhood*. It is published twice a year, July and January, at a cost of $3.25 per issue. It is oriented toward personal experience narratives and includes basic information about organizations congenial to family-centered maternity care. Also included are book lists. (Address: P.O. Box 184, Ridgway, Colorado 81432).

The Practicing Midwife is a newsletter which emerged from the January, 1977, First International Conference of Practicing Midwives, in El Paso, Texas. This new publication is intended to become a source of midwife statistics, a forum to share information and publicize conferences and news of midwifery. It will advertise available aids in midwife continuing training and serve as a clearinghouse for audio-visual materials. The newsletter issues from The Farm. Address: The Practicing Midwife, c/o Mildred Tassone and Edine Frohman, 156 Drakes Lane, Summertown, Tennessee, 38483.

For children

As we change in our ideas about birth, we change and determine in part how our children see it. Parents expecting a second or subsequent child confront the need to present the pregnancy, the birth, and the new sibling to the child or children who are already part of the family. Often a choice of home delivery enhances for other children the physical reality of birth, whether or not the children actually watch the delivery.

Although talk is obviously the first way to prepare with children, the various media have some offerings as well.

Books I describe here were selected if they met all the following criteria: (1) my daughter and four other eight-year-olds like them and have given me a positive report of them; (2) the proprietors of Great Brown Owl, a store selling exclusively children's books, enthusiastically recommend them; (3) a sex-educator I know recommends them; and (4) I like them. These books are of two sorts—those that help prepare children for a new baby in the family, and those that explain the processes of reproduction, pregnancy, and birth itself.

Among these, *Wind Rose,* by Crescent Dragonwagon, deserves special mention as an indicator of how changes in our experience of childbirth begin to appear in children's media and begin to prepare our children for their reproductive lives. *Wind Rose* is the story a mother tells her young daughter of the daughter's birth at home. The mother starts her story with the night they conceived Wind Rose, then describes the time of waiting through pregnancy:

. . . all the time we wondered and wondered
who is this person coming
growing   turning   floating   swimming
deep, deep inside.

The description of the birthing is particularly nice. Contractions are referred to as the belly "flexing." The birth is at home, and it is the mother and father together doing it, breathing together. The midwife arrives, Beulah, a wonderful warm big woman, who helps mothers and fathers.

Then suddenly I pushed,
I had to push I had to push,
I scrunched with this hard work of pushing.
The hole you came out of me through
was a stretching, burning circle.

The midwife has Wind Rose's mother stop pushing, to ease the baby out, and out she slips, "a strange and glistening slick fish-baby."

For all the poetry and simplicity of the language, and the lovely soft drawings, this is an accurate picture of birth, natural and real as it could be, and I am delighted that such a fine book exists.

Other books that prepare children for a new sibling include *Peter's Chair,* by Ezra Jack Keats; *The Knee Baby,* by Mary Jarrell (wife of the American poet and critic Randall Jarrell); *Go and Hush the Baby,* by Betsy Byars; and *That New Baby,* by Sara Bonnett Stein (this title is part of a series called *Open Family,* published by Walker and Co.). Nilsson's *A Child Is Born,* with its truly amazing photographs, is described in the Bibliography.

Among the books that explain reproduction to youngsters, *The Kids' Own XYZ of Love and Sex,* by Siv Widerberg, is a paperback my eight-year-old is reading now. She and her girlfriends peruse this book intently with exclamations of surprise and "Oh, yuk!"—inimitable. They also like Peter Mayle's *"Where Did I Come From?"* with its humorous drawings, and *Wind Rose.* Other recommended books: *Becoming,* by Eleanor Faison; and *Gabriel's Very First Birthday* (no author given; Pacific Pipeline Publishers).

It is heartening to see such well-written and well-illustrated books for children with themes such as the retarded child, adoption, and single-parent families, as well as the reproduction and birthing themes.

Television, too, has made an effort to present birth to kids. Twice in recent months in this (Philadelphia) area, ABC-TV aired an after-school special, "My Mom's Having a Baby," written by two women. The effort is a good one: to show birth and to present the feelings of the older child as he learns about pregnancy, labor, and delivery.

The hospital birth sequence in this movie is unclear at times. Everyone in it is draped and masked; there is an instrument being used but not explained (forceps, presumably—I couldn't really tell, and my daughter was quite concerned); some fairly vigorous pressure is applied to the woman's abdomen, too, which could confuse a child unless it were explained, which it wasn't. Also, since the woman had had a spinal, she did the pushing as instructed, not as prompted by signals from her own body. My response was to wish for a more strenuous and clear birth sequence.

The best presentation of birth sequences I have seen on television, for adults or for children, is the National Educational Television show called "Giving Birth," which I describe in the preceding section. I think a child would be relieved to see and understand the last of the four births in that program: the labor is hard work, but you can see exactly how it happens, and the unmitigated joy of the couple and the midwife afterward is gratifying to watch, for anybody.

7

Glossary of Terms

In this glossary of terms I have included words and concepts used in *The Birth Primer* and a selection of terms found in other basic books about childbirth. The Index to this book will lead you to further information about most of the entries that follow.

Abruptio placenta is the premature detachment of the placenta from the uterine wall (abruptio means a breaking off). Sometimes the condition is called placental abruption.

Accoucheur is a French word meaning midwife or obstetrician, one who attends a woman in labor.

Acidosis is a metabolic imbalance from the accumulation of excessive acid (or from a lack of base) in the body.

Afterbirth is made up of the placenta and the membranes associated with it when they are expelled after the baby is born.

After-pains occur as the uterus contracts after birth; these are like labor contractions. Almost unnoticeable after a first birth, after pains become more severe with each birth, as the work of the uterus to regain its normal size becomes increasingly difficult.

Amnesic drugs are for forgetfulness of pain. When such a drug is used during labor, it usually occurs in combination with the less potent analgesics. Scopolamine is an amnesic that is sometimes administered during labor.

Amniocentesis is the process of withdrawing some amniotic fluid from the bag of waters, or amniotic sac, by inserting a needle through the abdomen and uterine wall. This technique originally was used to monitor Rh-sensitive women but now is increasingly employed to check for a number of hereditary disorders such as hemophilia and Down's syndrome.

Amnion is the inner one of the two membranes that surround the fetus to form the bag of waters, or amniotic sac. The other membrane is called the chorion.

Amniotic fluid is the transparent fluid which fills the amniotic sac. The fluid serves the fetus in many ways: it maintains an even temperature in the womb; it allows the fetus to move easily and protects her from injury; and it prevents the amnion from sticking to the skin of the fetus. It is constantly being replenished. At birth there is usually about 500 to 1000 ml of amniotic fluid.

Amniotic sac is the transparent bag composed of two membranes and containing the amniotic fluid. The fetus is surrounded by the fluid-filled sac, which expands as the fetus grows. It is also called the bag of waters.

Amniotomy is the labor-inducing or labor-stimulating procedure in which the amniotic sac is artificially ruptured by a sharp instrument introduced through the birth canal and the partly dilated cervix.

Analgesic, from the Green *an*, meaning not, and *algesis*, meaning pain, is the class of drugs that relieve pain without causing loss of consciousness. Analgesics administered during labor include Demerol, methadone, and Nisentil.

Anesthesia is insensibility, loss of sensation, either general, regional, or local; this condition is produced by anesthetic agents.

Anesthetic agents used during labor may be general (to produce unconsciousness), regional (to numb a specific nerve, as in epidural block or saddle block), or local (to deaden pain in a specific small area).

Anoxia is a lack or absence of oxygen; this condition sometimes occurs in newborns.

Ante-natal means before birth.

Antiseptic preparations inhibit the growth of bacteria but do not necessarily kill them. Boric acid and alcohol are commonly used antiseptics.

Apgar score, developed by Dr. Virginia Apgar, an American anesthesiologist, is an assessment of the health of a baby one minute after birth and five minutes after birth. Included in this calculation are heart rate, muscle tone, respiratory effort, reflex irritability, and skin color.

Asphyxia, a condition characterized by anoxia, a feeling of suffocation, and coma, may occur in the newborn.

Aspiration is the act of sucking in; aspiration of meconium is a danger for the fetus in distress.

Aspiration pneumonia is pneumonia caused by the breathing in of foreign substances; this complication occurs sometimes in the birth of a fetus in distress who fills his lungs before being born, and takes in amniotic fluid and meconium.

Atony is absence of or lack of tone in a muscle; in the uterus, atony signifies a degree of inertia.

Bag of waters is synonymous with amniotic sac.

Barbiturate drugs come from barbituric acid and are sometimes given to women in labor to make them sleep. Common barbiturates include Nembutal and Seconal. These drugs can have a negative effect on the fetus.

Birth canal, as the name indicates, is the channel through which the fetus passes to enter the world. It is synonymous with the vagina; sometimes the cervix is included in descriptions of this passageway.

Blood pressure refers to the pressure of the blood on the walls of the arteries. It is divided into two parts: maximum pressure, or systolic pressure, occurs when the left ventricle of the heart contracts; minimum pressure, or diastolic pressure, occurs when the ventricle dilates. High blood pressure is called hypertension; low blood pressure is hypotension. Blood pressure must be monitored carefully during labors in which anesthetic agents or labor-stimulating hormones are used.

Bloody show, or show, is the passing of the mucous plug that has corked the cervix closed during pregnancy. Often the mucus is flecked with blood. Bloody show usually occurs just prior to labor and sometimes throughout the first stage. Sometimes the term show or bloody show refers to the mucous plug itself.

Bonding is the phenomenon of attachment-forming between mother and offspring that occurs in the sensitive period immediately following birth. This process occurs through sight, touch, and smell. Medications given to the woman in labor can interfere with the process.

Brachycardia is synonymous with bradycardia.

Bradycardia, from the Greek words meaning slow (*bradys*) and heart (*kardia*), means abnormal slowness of the heartbeat. Bradycardia can occur particularly during the second half of labor if a woman lies flat on her back.

Braxton-Hicks contractions are painless, intermittent uterine contractions, named for an English gynecologist of the nineteenth century. They occur throughout pregnancy and especially toward the end, when they are helping to begin the softening and taking up of the sides of the cervix.

Breech delivery occurs when the baby's buttocks (his breech) or feet come out first.

Breech position describes the placement of the fetus in a breech delivery; the buttocks, or feet, come out first instead of the head.

Bucally means by mouth, often referring to the administration of medication.

Caesarean section is birth via surgical incision of the abdomen and the uterus. The operation is performed when natural passage through the birth canal is impossible: for example, if the mother's pelvis is too small to accommodate the baby's head size; if the umbilical cord prolapses; if there is hemorrhage from placenta previa or abruptio placenta; or if severe fetal distress is present. So named, it is said, because Julius Caesar may have been delivered in this way. Also spelled Cesarean; also called C-section.

Cardiopulmonary resuscitation, abbreviated CPR, is emergency resuscitation (e.g., of the neonate) through stimulation of heart and lungs.

Catching a baby is what the attendant does in labor; delivering is the mother's job.

Catheter, a tube for withdrawing fluid from the body, is sometimes used to drain urine from the bladder in pregnant women so that the descent of the fetus is not blocked by a full bladder.

Caudal block is a regional anesthetic procedure in which the drug is injected at the base of the spine during the first stage of labor and subsequently, if necessary. *Cauda* is the Latin word for tail.

Cephalopelvic disproportion means that the baby's head (Greek *kephalos* = head) is too large to pass through the mother's pelvis. Caesarean section may be necessary. Abbreviated CPD.

Cerebrospinal fluid, or CSF, is contained in the brain and spinal cord. It may be withdrawn by needle for examination to determine the presence of certain neurologic disorders. The headache that follows spinal anesthesia is thought to be caused by leakage of CSF at the site of the injection.

Cervix is the Latin word for neck. The *cervix uteri* is the lower, narrow end of the uterus, its opening into the birth canal. When we talk about being x-centimeters dilated, we are referring to the dilation or opening up of the cervix.

Childbed fever is synonymous with puerperal fever.

Chloroform was one of the first general anesthetics to be discovered. It is rarely used today during labor.

Chorion is the outer of the two membranes that compose the amniotic sac.

Cleansing breath is part of the breathing exercises practiced in Lamaze and other childbirth preparation courses. A cleansing breath is a deep breath. One is done at the beginning of each contraction, and one at the end, to assure the mother and fetus adequate oxygen in the stress of labor.

Colostrum, the first breast milk, is a thin yellowish fluid that begins to be secreted by the breasts after about the nineteenth week of pregnancy. It is full of the antibodies needed especially by a premature baby, and is similarly rich in protein, minerals, vitamin A, and nitrogen.

Conduction anesthetic is synonymous with regional anesthetic.

Contractions are shortenings or tensings of a muscle. The uterus experiences a series of these tensings to open the cavity and then to push out the fetus.

Cord prolapse occurs when the umbilical cord slips down into the vaginal canal before the fetus does. Fetal oxygen supply is threatened, and the mother's abdomen must be kept high to prevent further slipping. This problem usually requires Caesarean section.

Crowning is that amazing moment when the baby's head (or crown) visibly causes the perineum to bulge; birth is imminent.

Delivering a baby is what the woman does in childbirth; catching is the job of the attendant (doctor, midwife, whoever).

Delivery begins with the second stage of labor, when the cervix is fully dilated and the fetus can start to descend the birth canal; it ends with the birth. Delivery is considered part of labor.

Demerol, a trademark for meperidine or pethidine, is a narcotic that may be administered during labor to make the mother relax or doze off. Demerol is a synthetic morphine.

Diabetes is a disorder of sugar metabolism; it requires close monitoring during pregnancy. The diabetic woman's insulin requirements may change frequently during pregnancy and immediately after delivery, and the incidence of premature births in this group is high.

Diaphragm, from the Greek word meaning partition or barrier, is the muscular sheet that separates the abdominal cavity from the chest cavity. Breathing exercises used during labor call for diaphragmatic control.

Dilatation, or the opening up of the cervix, is the work of the first stage of labor.

Dilation, the opening up of the cervix, is generally used synonymously with dilatation.

Diuretic agents stimulate urination.

Dystocia means difficult labor.

Eclampsia consists of convulsions and coma; it is an advanced stage of toxemia that may occur during pregnancy or labor.

Edema means swelling.

Effacement is the gradual flattening of or taking up of the sides of the cervix that occurs during early labor, along with or just before dilatation.

Effleurage, a kind of massage taught first in the Lamaze method, is one of the relaxing techniques used by the laboring woman or labor coach. The abdomen is gently massaged with the fingertips, up from the base of the abdomen in a circle as you inhale, and back down again on the exhale. Corn starch or talcum powder may be rubbed on the abdomen to prevent discomfort from friction.

Embryo, from the Greek *en*, meaning in, and *bruein*, meaning to grow, is the name for the developing human from conception to the end of the second month, at which time he is called a fetus.

Endometrium, from the Greek *endo*, meaning within, and *metra*, meaning womb, refers to the membranous lining of the uterus, in which the fertilized egg matures. If fertilization does not occur, most of the endometrium is sloughed off; this is menstruation.

Enema, an injection of liquid into the rectum, is often part of the hospital preparation for labor. In addition to emptying the rectum, it stimulates uterine contractions.

Epidural block is a form of regional anesthetic injected into the back and administered continuously via a catheter.

Episiotomy is a surgical cut of the perineum to make more room at the vaginal opening and thus prevent possibly ragged tearing when the baby's head emerges. Episiotomies are done routinely in hospital delivery.

Ergot, the main ingredient in the various oxytocics, is a fungus which grows on rye plants. Used for labor stimulation for eons by mid-wives, it was isolated in the late sixteenth century by researchers at a European university.

Ether, one of the earliest forms of general anesthetic to be discovered, is not much used for delivery anymore, because it slows down labor, has a negative effect on the baby, and may be fatal to the mother if she inhales too much of it.

Expulsion stage is synonymous with the second stage of labor.

External version is the manipulation of the fetal position (usually in cases of transverse lie) from outside the mother's body by alternate stroking and pushing motions on her abdomen.

Fetal heart monitor is a machine which measures and reports the rate of heartbeat of the fetus. Developed in the 1950s, it has two aspects, external (a device is belted on the woman's abdomen) and internal (an electrode is fastened to the fetal scalp after partial dilation has occurred). A pressure gauge to record the incidence of contractions can also be strapped on externally.

Fetus is the term used for the developing person from the end of the second month in utero until it is completely outside the mother's body.

First stage of labor begins at the onset of strong uterine contractions and lasts until the cervix is completely dilated. The three parts of first-stage labor are early (up to 5 cm), active (5 cm to 8 cm), and transition (8 cm to 10 cm).

Fontanelle is the space at the junction of sutures in the skull of the infant. This French word means little fountain, and it was so named because the pulsation that can be felt there was assumed to be the bubbling of a small fountain of blood, before the circulation of the blood was understood.

Footling breech is a breech delivery in which the feet of the baby present first.

Forceps, invented in the sixteenth century, is an instrument resembling a pair of ice tongs that is sometimes used to pull the baby out. Forceps delivery may be high, mid, or low, depending on how far up the birth canal the instrument must be inserted; high-forceps deliveries are now rare.

Full-term refers to a pregnancy that lasts a full 280 days.

Fundus is the portion of any organ that is farthest from its opening; thus the fundus of the uterus is the uppermost part, where the contracting movement begins.

General anesthetic agents cause unconsciousness and deaden the entire body to pain.

Gynecology comes from the Greek *gyne,* meaning woman, and *logos,* meaning to study. This branch of medicine deals with all aspects of the female genital tract.

Hallucinogenic drugs cause you to perceive things that are not objectively present. Scopolamine is a hallucinogen sometimes used during labor.

Hemorrhage is excessive bleeding. Placenta previa and abruptio placenta cause prepartum hemorrhage; postpartum hemorrhage may be caused by abnormal relaxation of the uterine muscles, retained placenta, or lacerations in the birth canal.

High-forceps delivery refers to the depth to which the forceps are placed inside the mother to reach the baby. This is the most dangerous type of delivery, since the baby must be pulled over a long distance; it is rare nowadays.

Hormone comes from the Greek word meaning to arouse to action. These chemicals are produced in the endocrine glands of the body and carried by the blood or other bodily fluid to act upon a specific organ or cells. Estrogen and progesterone are hormones produced by the ovaries. Oxytocin is the hormone which stimulates uterine contractions.

Hyaline membrane disease, also known as respiratory distress syndrome (RDS), is a respiratory disease that sometimes affects premature infants.

Hyper- is the prefix from the Greek meaning over, or excessive.

Hypertension means high blood pressure. Use of the contraceptive pill raises the blood pressure, sometimes to hypertensive levels; so does induction of labor. Women with high blood pressure are at risk in labor.

Hyperventilation is abnormally rapidly breathing resulting in dizziness. It can occur in the laboring woman if her quick breathing causes an imbalance of oxygen and carbon dioxide.

Hypo- is the prefix from the Greek meaning under, or lacking in.

Hypodermic refers to injections that are administered into the tissues under the skin, or subcutaneously. Sometimes the syringe used for the injection is called a hypodermic.

Hypotension means abnormally low blood pressure, which may develop in the mother as a result of regional anesthesia.

Hypoxia occurs when the fetus is not getting enough oxygen. The fetal heart monitor can detect hypoxia, which is also called acute fetal distress.

Hysteria comes from the Greek *hustera,* meaning uterus; thus the condition of hysteria ("excessive emotionality") is named after the woman's organs of reproduction, and a hysterectomy was believed to remove the cause of hysterics.

Immature describes the stage of development of systems in the premature baby, in particular his respiration.

Immunoglobulin is a substance produced by the body to protect it from infection. The mother's immunoglobulins cross the placenta and protect the fetus. Immunoglobulins are also present in colostrum and may provide immunity for the infant's intestinal tract.

In utero means, literally, in the uterus (Latin).

Induction of labor means that the uterus is artificially stimulated to contract, thus speeding up the first stage of labor. This is done by rupturing the bag of waters and/or by administering the synthetic hormone Pitocin.

Inhalants are drugs that are taken by being breathed in through the mouth or nose. General anesthetics are often given in inhalant form.

Intramuscular injections are administered into muscle tissue.

Intravenous (I.V.) means injected into the veins. This is the route for most types of continuous therapy, such as replacement of fluids. Labor-stimulating hormones are often given I.V.

Involution is the returning of the uterus to its pre-pregnant size and shape. This process begins with contractions immediately after birth, and may take two to four weeks.

Labor encompasses the entire process of pushing the fetus from the uterus into the outside world; it means, of course, work.

Laceration is a term meaning a tear or a rip in the flesh.

Lay midwife is a midwife who has received training from direct experience in attending women in labor, usually first as an apprentice, rather than through a medical course of study.

Lie is synonymous with presentation, as in transverse lie of a fetus.

Lightening means that the fetus has descended into the pelvic cavity in preparation of delivery. It usually happens about two weeks before the beginning of labor in primaparas (later in subsequent labors) and is so called because of the characteristic feeling of a decrease in pressure on the organs of the upper abdomen.

Lithotomy position is the familiar "gynecologist's office" position—you lie flat on your back, with legs elevated and spread and feet in stirrups. This is a common position for delivery but not the best one, since it is impossible to push effectively while lying down; gravity is not helping you, as it would if you were squatting.

"Little" spinal is another name for the regional anesthetic called saddle block.

Local anesthetic means that only a small, specific area of the body is numbed, as when the perineum is anesthetized for the repair of an episiotomy.

Lochia, a plural term, names discharge from the placental site on the uterine wall after birth; the lochia begin dark red and gradually over two weeks or so after birth reduce in amount and lighten in color.

Low birth weight infants weigh at birth less than 2500 grams, or 5 lbs. 8 oz.

Meconium is the first excretion by the newborn. It is composed of the baby's intestinal contents plus some amniotic fluid, and it is greenish-black. Premature expulsion by the fetus of meconium into the amniotic fluid is called meconium staining and is a signal of distress.

Menstruation comes from the Latin word *mensis,* which mean month. It refers to the uterine bleeding that occurs every month during the reproductive life of a woman when she is not pregnant. If pregnancy occurs, this blood forms the lining of the uterus, in which the fertilized egg grows; if pregnancy does not occur, the lining is not needed and thus is sloughed off.

Meperidine is the chemical name for Demerol, a narcotic analgesic. In England it is called Pethidine.

Midwife is the title given to people who are trained to assist in childbirth. The word derives from the Old English, meaning "with the woman."

Morphine, a narcotic, is the active ingredient of opium and is used as an analgesic.

Multipara means a woman giving birth for the second or subsequent time; often abbreviated multip. From the Latin *multi,* meaning many, and the verb *parere,* to give birth.

Narcotic comes from the Greek word meaning to benumb. These drugs dull the senses, produce stupor, or induce sleep, and they can become addictive. Demerol is one of the narcotics most commonly given in labor.

Nembutal, a trademark for pentobarbital, is a barbiturate. This drug has been used to produce sleep in laboring mothers, but it is dangerous to the fetus because it decreases fetal respiration.

Neonate means a newborn baby.

Neonatology is the branch of medicine dealing with the care of the newborn, or neonate. This field of study overlaps with perinatology; both are branches of pediatrics.

Nurse-midwife is a midwife who has trained first as a nurse and then has gone on to study midwifery in a special program of some 12 to 24 months. A nurse-midwife usually practices on the staff of a maternity center; sometimes in a hospital; almost never, at this time, independently.

Obstetrics is the branch of medicine that deals with pregnancy, labor, and birth. Obstetrics comes from the Latin word for midwife, *obstetrix*, which means "she who stands by."

Occiput means the back of the head.

Oxytocics are labor stimulants.

Oxytocin is a hormone which speeds up labor by stimulating contractions of the uterus. Pitocin is a trademark for synthetic oxytocin.

Paracervical block is an anesthetic used during the active phase of first-stage labor. A local anesthetic is injected at the junction of the vagina and cervix, and a catheter may be placed for continuous administration of the anesthetic. There are usually no side effects for the mother, but the fetus may experience bradycardia, and there is a risk of respiratory depression in both fetus and neonate.

Parturient, from the Latin *parturitio*, means to be giving birth, or refers to a woman in labor.

Parturition is the act of giving birth.

Pelvic floor is another name for the perineum, the bottom of the pelvic basin, the area between the vulva and the anus.

Pelvis comes from the Greek *pyelos*, meaning an oblong trough or basin. This is the area bounded on either side and in front by the hipbones and in back by the base of the spine.

Perinatal describes the period of time just before, during, and just after birth.

Perinatology, from the Greek *peri*, meaning around, and the Latin *natus*, meaning born, is the branch of medicine dealing with the care of the newborn to about one to four weeks after birth.

Perineum is the floor of the pelvis, also called the pelvic diaphragm. The external part of the perineum is the area between the anus and the vaginal opening. It is the perineum that is cut in an episiotomy.

Pitocin is a trademark for synthetic oxytocin.

Pituitary gland is the major endocrine gland; it regulates the functions of many of the other glands such as the thyroid and the gonads. Oxytocin, the hormone that induces uterine contractions, is stored in the pituitary. Also called the hypophysis.

Placenta, from the Latin meaning a flat cake, is the organ which communicates between mother and fetus, via the umbilical cord. It is through the placenta that the fetus receives nourishment and oxygen and discards waste. About one half hour after the baby is born, the placenta is expelled; this is called third-stage labor, or the expulsion of the afterbirth.

Placenta previa is a condition in which the placenta lies over the cervix, rather than high up in the uterus. The primary symptom is painless bleeding, which usually develops during the final trimester. Placenta previa is classified as complete, partial, or marginal, depending on how much of the cervix is covered. For complete or partial placenta previa, Caesarean section is usually necessary, but in marginal cases normal delivery is sometimes possible.

Pneumonia is inflammation of the lungs. In the newborn it may be the result of early rupture of the membranes, prolonged labor, aspiration of fluid and meconium during birth, or infection.

Podalic version is a manipulation of fetal position by the accoucheur, specifically, the bringing of the legs or buttocks down into the pelvis. This very difficult and very delicate type of maneuver is usually used only in cases of transverse lie where the membrane has not ruptured or in delivering a second twin.

Posterior presentation refers to the fetal position in which the unborn is facing the mother's front instead of her back, as is most usual (anterior). Posterior presentation causes back pain in the mother during labor; often the fetus turns during labor and faces the other way.

Postmature refers to infants of whom the placenta has ceased to function properly. A baby born two weeks or more after the expected time may be in this condition.

Postpartum means after the birth.

Pre-eclampsia is a toxemia of pregnancy that occurs in the third trimester. The main symptoms are hypertension, weight gain, edema, and the presence of protein in the urine. The cause of this poisoning is unknown.

Premature refers to any live infant born at less than 38 weeks' gestation, that is less than 38 weeks since the mother's last menstruation began. Also called pre-term. Since premature babies are usually low birth weight, and since gestational age is notoriously hard to compute, the definition for low birth weight is often used (that is, an infant born weighing less than 2500 grams, or 5 lb. 8 oz.) for prematurity.

Prepping is the common term for preparation of the mother for labor and delivery at the hospital, specifically referring to the shaving of the pubic hair.

Present (verb) means to show, and refers to the appearance of the first part (called the presenting part) of the fetus at delivery, usually the head.

Presentation means lie of the fetus; that is, it refers to the part of the fetus that will present itself first. In vertex presentations, the most common position (95% of labors), the baby is head down. Breech presentations, where the rear or the feet present first, are much less common. Face and brow presentations are rarer still. A transverse lie, in which the fetus is not longitudinal at all but crosswise, is extremely infrequent, and cannot be delivered vaginally.

Primigravida is a woman who is pregnant for the first time; from the Latin *gravida,* meaning heavy, and *prima,* meaning first.

Primipara means a woman giving birth for the first time; often abbreviated primap. From the Latin verb *parere,* to give birth.

Prolapse means the falling of an organ or part, as in cord prolapse or prolapse of the uterus.

Proteinuria, the presence of protein in the urine, is one of the symptoms of eclampsia.

Psychoprophylaxis comes from the Greek words for mind (*psyche*) and to protect (*prophylassein*). It encompasses the techniques of physical and mental preparation for birth—breathing exercises, instruction in labor and delivery—used to help the mother experience childbirth with the greatest awareness and the least amount of pain. It was Dr. Lamaze who brought the term into popular usage.

Pudendal block is a regional anesthetic technique that numbs the pudendal nerve and thus all of the mother's external genital area. It is used during second- and third-stage labor and for episiotomy repair.

Pudendum (plural, pudenda) refers to the external genital organs, especially of the female, from the Latin verb *pudere,* meaning to be ashamed.

Puerpera is a woman in labor or recently delivered. From the Latin *puer,* meaning child, and *parere,* to bring forth, give birth to.

Puerperal fever is an infection of the birth canal caused by the presence of bacteria. Also known as puerperal sepsis, puerperal septicemia, and childbed fever, this disease was a great killer of new mothers before the importance of absolute cleanliness in hospitals was recognized.

Puerperium is the six-week period following delivery, during which the pelvic organs return to their normal positions, and infant feeding is established.

Regional anesthetic procedures block specific nerves so that the sensory message from the area supplied by the nerve does not reach the brain. All the "blocks"—pudendal, caudal, epidural, etc.—are forms of regional anesthetic.

Respiratory distress syndrome, abbreviated RDS, afflicts premature babies especially; it is also called hyaline membrane disease.

Rh factor stands for rhesus factor, a substance discovered through experimentation with rhesus monkeys. This substance is present in the blood of most people; people containing it are called Rh-positive (Rh +), and those lacking it are called Rh-negative (Rh -). If the mother is Rh - and the father is Rh +, the baby in utero is usually (but not always) Rh-positive. When a positive baby is inside a negative mother, some of the baby's blood can get into the mother; she responds to this by making antibodies in her blood that can hurt her baby and future babies. Since this transference of blood usually happens at the time of delivery, an injection after birth can prevent nearly every sensitization of the Rh-negative mother by delivery of an Rh-positive baby.

Rooming-in is the practice of having the baby stay in the room with the mother in the hospital for all or most of the day and sometimes for the night as well.

Saddle block is a regional anesthetic for the lower part of the spine. It is so named because it numbs the area that comes in contact with a saddle when riding horseback—buttocks, perineum, and inner thighs. Like other regional blocks, this one may cause low blood pressure in the mother.

Scopolamine is an amnesic and hallucinogenic drug that is used with sedatives to induce what is known as "twilight sleep" in the mother. There is no numbing as in anesthesia and analgesia: the woman feels all sensations in a half-sleep state, but afterwards does not consciously remember anything.

Seconal is a trademark for a barbiturate that causes sleep during labor. Like the other barbiturates, this one crosses the placental barrier and can have a negative effect on fetal respiration.

Second stage of labor begins when the cervix is fully dilated and ends when the baby is born.

Sedative agents calm the patient. Included in this category are the barbiturates, such as Seconal and Nembutal, although in high doses barbiturates produce sleep rather than mere sedation. Sedatives are usually given orally, during the early stages of labor.

Sepsis, a Greek word meaning decay, refers to poisoning caused by bacterial infection, as of the genitals during labor or immediately afterward.

Show is synonymous with bloody show.

Sonography is a technique for visualizing the body's internal structures by the reflection of sound waves. Safer than x-rays because no harmful radiation is involved, this technique is used to detect the presence of twins or of placenta previa, to assess fetal development, and for many other diagnostic purposes.

Spinal block is the numbing of the lower regions of the body by injection of local anesthetic into the area around the spinal cord, called the subarachnoid space. The two main types of spinal block for vaginal delivery are the low spinal and the saddle block. For Caesarean section, the injection is made higher up in the spine. One complication of spinal anesthesia is low blood pressure in the mother.

Spontaneous abortion refers to expulsion of the fetus due to natural causes, in contrast to abortion that is induced deliberately. In most cases the cause of spontaneous abortion is not known.

Spontaneous delivery is delivery without forceps.

Standing orders refer to a doctor's routine use of medicines and procedures. An obstetrician sometimes leaves blanket instructions for particular substances or procedures to be administered to his patients in labor during his absence.

Station is a method of gauging the extent of engagement of the baby's presenting part in the pelvis; normal range is from minus one to plus one. With a baby in vertex presentation, at minus one station, the head is not deeply engaged in the cervical opening; at zero station, the head is level with the ischial spines, bones in the pelvis; at plus one station the baby's head has begun to descend into the birth canal.

Sucking reflex is a response with which all babies are born. When a newborn's lips are stimulated, her jaws and mouth know how to suck.

Term refers to the natural duration of pregnancy, 280 days.

Third stage of labor consists of delivery of the placenta and membranes, which usually takes place within 30 to 45 minutes after the baby is born; also referred to as the expulsion of the afterbirth.

Toxemia means poisoning by bacterial infection. Toxemia of pregnancy may lead to pre-eclampsia and eclampsia.

Tranquilizers are used during labor to help the mother relax between contractions. These drugs are milder than many other analgesics and usually do not cause sleep. Valium and Sparine are trademarks for commonly used tranquilizers.

Transition is the final, most difficult, and shortest phase of first-stage labor. During transition, the cervix opens from 8 centimeters' dilation to the full 10 centimeters. Contractions are intense, and the baby's head moves into the birth canal. Thus the transition is from the work of dilation to the work of pushing out the baby.

Transverse lie means that the back or shoulder of the fetus is across the opening of the birth canal. A fetus lying transverse must turn or be turned to be born vaginally; Caesarean section is otherwise the method of delivery. About 1% of babies remain transverse. This presentation is more common in multiparas and in premature labors.

Trimester means a three-month period. Pregnancy is divided into three trimesters, each of 13 + weeks and each with its own characteristics and risks.

Twilight sleep refers to the state induced during labor by the administration of the amnesic scopolamine.

Umbilical cord, the lifeline of the fetus, is attached to the abdomen of the fetus and to the placenta. It is through this cord that the fetus passes wastes to the mother and receives nutrients and oxygen from her.

Umbilicus is the scar or mark left on the baby where the umbilical cord was cut; the navel.

Uterine inertia means lack of progress in labor such that the doctor or midwife may consider intervention. The amount of time that must elapse before a state of inertia is judged to exist is not consistently specified by obstetricians, although it is greater for the primapara than for the multipara.

Uterus is the hollow muscular organ in which the fetus develops; also known as the womb.

Vacuum extraction is the technique developed in Sweden (and more popular in Europe than here) to aid in the removal of the fetus from the birth canal.

Vagina is the birth canal; it extends from the vulva to the cervix. The Latin word vagina means sheath, as of a sword.

Vernix is the waxy or cheesy substance that covers and protects the skin of the fetus while it is in the uterus.

Version is the turning around of the fetus while in the uterus in order to place it in a more favorable position of delivery. To accomplish external version, the doctor coaxes the fetus into a better position by manipulation of the mother's abdomen. In internal podalic version, a rare occurrence, the attendant reaches up through the birth canal, through the opened cervix, and grabs the the feet of the fetus lying transverse, thus transforming the presentation to a footling breech delivery.

Vertex means the top of the head. The most common type of delivery is the vertex presentation, in which the top of the fetal head emerges first.

Vulva comprises all of the female external genitalia: the labia majora, labia minora, clitoris, and the opening of the vagina.

Water is used synonymously with amniotic fluid. The amniotic sac is often called the bag of waters; thus the amniotic fluid is the water.

8

Annotated Bibliography

The main purpose of this bibliography is to list and describe popular childbirth books on the market today. Classic childbirth books and selected works of related interest are also included. Prices are for paperback editions unless otherwise indicated. The Bibliography also includes articles and textbooks that I have referred to in the chapters. Books especially for children and publications (newsletters, pamphlets, etc.) issued by the various childbirth organizations are described in Chapter 6.

Apgar, Virginia, M.D., and Joan Beck. *Is My Baby All Right?* New York: Pocket Books, 1974. $1.95. First published by Simon & Schuster, Inc., 1972. A description of the things that can go wrong metabolically and genetically and during labor and birth, which can damage a baby. The language is technical enough to be correct but is accessible to all; though the topics are often tragic, the treatment given by Dr. Apgar and Ms. Beck manages to be reassuring. A valuable contribution.

Arms, Suzanne, and John Arms. *A Season to Be Born*. New York: Harper & Row, Publishers, Inc., Harper Colophon Books, 1973. $3.50 A lovely, personal book of photographs and reflections by the woman who went on to write *Immaculate Deception*. The subject is her own first pregnancy and the birth of her daughter, in the local hospital, with her husband as coach and companion.

Arms, Suzanne. *Immaculate Deception: A New Look at Women and Childbirth in America*. Boston: Houghton Mifflin Co., 1975. $6.50. Bantam Books edition, with a foreword by Leboyer, 1977. $2.50. Very important exploration of the warping of childbirth in recent years in America. Excellent section on midwives, extremely good accounts of personal experiences. Wide-ranging, influential. This work is a groundbreaker, passionate and pointed; Arms' all-out condemnation of American hospital birth seems excessive at times, but her warnings and discoveries continue to serve us well.

Ashdown-Sharp, Patricia. *A Guide to Pregnancy and Parenthood for Women on Their Own*. New York: Vintage Books, a division of Random House, 1977. $3.95. A practical guide; how to know whether or not you're pregnant, how to arrange adoption, how to arrange for birth or for abortion. The author has valuable suggestions to offer about finding financial and emotional assistance.

Banet, Barbara Edwards, and Mary Lou Rozdilsky. *What Now? A Handbook for New Parents*. New York: Charles Scribner's Sons, 1975. Cloth, $7.95. A book of sensible guidelines, readable and reassuring; it includes discussions of the role of the father, of lifestyle alternatives for mothers, and of sexuality after the birth.

A Barefoot Doctor's Manual: The American Translation of the Official Chinese Paramedical Manual. Philadelphia: Running Press, 1977. $5.95. A fascinating manual of medicine as practiced by paramedical workers in China. It includes a section on medicinal plants, an introduction to diagnostic techniques, folk treatments, and a large chapter on birth control and delivery of babies.

Barker-Benfield, Ben. *The Horrors of the Half-Known Life: Male Attitudes Toward Women and Sexuality in Nineteenth-Century America*. New York: Harper & Row, Publishers, Inc., Harper Colophon Books, 1976. $4.50. A scholarly work, containing valuable background material about midwives and the suppression of their work.

Bean, Constance A. *Labor & Delivery: An Observer's Diary*. Garden City, New York: Doubleday & Co., Inc., 1977. Cloth, $7.95. A firsthand account of the kinds of choices available today in childbirth; the diary approach, combined with Ms. Bean's extensive knowledge of the subject, gives this book a positive strength and the readability of a novel. She visited many kinds of facilities and reports vividly and sympathetically what she saw.

Bean, Constance A. *Methods of Childbirth*. Garden City, New York: Doubleday & Co., Inc., Dolphin Books Edition, 1974. $1.95. First published 1972. One of the basic information books, like a childbirth education class in itself. Covers drugs, role of fathers, breast feeding, relaxation and breathing preparation for birth; lacks an index.

Beck, Joan. *Effective Parenting*. New York: Simon & Schuster, Inc., 1976. Cloth, $8.95. Sound advice, relying on much of the latest information available from social scientists and educators about how best to navigate parenthood.

Bel Geddes, Joan. *How to Parent Alone*. New York: The Seabury Press, A Continuum Book, 1974. Cloth, $8.95. This book presents some good ideas about how to cope with this challenging experience.

Benson, Herbert, M.D. *The Relaxation Response*. New York: William Morrow & Co., Inc., 1975. Cloth, $5.95. Basic information about the value of relaxation techniques to general health; useful.

Benson, Ralph C., M.D. *Current Obstetric and Gynecologic Diagnosis and Treatment.* Los Altos, California: Lange Medical Publications, 1976. Cloth, $16.00. A standard obstetrical textbook, unnecessarily technical for the general reader. Benson does discuss "natural childbirth procedures," including preparation for birth, participation of the father, and less extensive use of drugs.

Bing, Elisabeth (Ed.). *The Adventure of Birth: Experiences in the Lamaze Method of Prepared Childbirth.* New York: Ace Books, A Division of Charter Communications, Inc., 1970. $1.25. In this book, Ms. Bing recounts the birth experiences of some of the many couples who have trained with her in the Lamaze method. The stories are immediate and fun to read.

Bing, Elisabeth. *Moving Through Pregnancy.* New York: Bobbs-Merrill Co., Inc., 1975. $4.50. Photographs of pregnant woman doing recommended exercises.

Bing, Elisabeth. *Six Practical Lessons for an Easier Childbirth.* New York: Bantam Books, Inc., 1973. $1.95. Originally published by Crosset & Dunlap, Inc., 1967. The Lamaze method, in step-by-step guide form. Fully illustrated, reassuring; a handy manual.

Birth Atlas. See under Maternity Center Association.

Birth and Family Journal. 110 El Camino Real, Berkeley, California, 94705. An important journal that covers many aspects of pregnancy, labor, birth, postpartum, and family life.

Boston Children's Medical Center. *Pregnancy, Birth & The Newborn Baby.* New York: Delacorte Press/Seymour Lawrence, 1971. Cloth, $14.95. A handsome book, but its main value is in the two preliminary essays, by Niles Newton and by Margaret Mead, on aspects of childbearing in a changing world. For such a cost, the text is rather brief on medical detail and tends not to consider nonmedical views.

Boston Women's Health Book Collective, Inc. *Our Bodies, Ourselves.* 2nd Edition. New York: Simon & Schuster, Inc., 1976. $4.95. Enormously popular and rightly so: this is the single most important book about women's health. It is available for clinics at reduced rates. First published as a large newsprint pamphlet in 1971, it has become a classic and a best-seller. Sections on pregnancy, birth, and postpartum are clear, medically correct, informative, supportive, and well written, like the rest of the book. The authors evaluate the available options from the point of view of consumers of health care, and they encourage us to do the same.

Bowlby, John. *Child Care and the Growth of Love.* 2nd Edition;

based by permission of the World Health Organization on the Report *Maternal Care and Mental Health,* by John Bowlby; abridged and edited by Margery Fry, with two new chapters by Mary D. Salter Ainsworth. Baltimore, Maryland: Penguin Books Inc., 1953; 2nd Edition, 1965. $1.25. Studies and speculations about the effects of deprivation of mothering on the growth and mental health of the child.

Bradley, Robert A., M.D. *Husband-Coached Childbirth.* Revised Edition. New York: Harper & Row, Publishers, Inc., 1974. Cloth, $6.95. First publsihed 1965. Useful information about full participation of the husband in the childbirth experience; the author, an obstetrician, has attended at more than 10,000 deliveries. His vocabulary is occasionally patronizing (the uterus is called the "baby box") but his method has widespread popularity, and the book is worth reading.

Brennan, Barbara, C.N.M., and Joan Rattner Heilman. *The Complete Book of Midwifery.* New York: E.P. Dutton & Co., Inc., 1977. $4.95. A fine description of the work of the modern nurse-midwife. Parent-centered childbirth is emphasized, along with the midwife's traditional protection of laboring women from unnecessary medical interference. The photographs are numerous and good. Hospital birth is the choice here; Brennan projects optimism about kinds of change hospitals are capable of. There is also historical material on midwifery.

Brewer, Gail, and Thomas Brewer, M.D. *What Every Pregnant Woman Should Know: The Truth About Diet and Drugs in Pregnancy.* New York: Random House, 1977. Cloth, $8.95. This book is written in basic language and is full of advice to pregnant women about how to safeguard their health and the health of their unborn. Dr. Thomas Brewer is the author of articles and a book on toxemia and its relation to nutrition.

Brewer Thomas, M.D. *Metabolic Toxemia of Late Pregnancy: A Disease of Malnutrition.* Springfield, Illinois: Charles C. Thomas, Publisher, 1966. Cloth, $8.50. Discovery of connection between nutrition and toxemias of pregnancy is presented here by the doctor who has most noticeably worked to fight this problem, and who also founded SPUN, Society for the Protection of the Unborn through Nutrition (see Chapter 6). Brewer gives explicit dietary advice.

Bricklin, Alice. *MotherLove: Natural Mothering, Birth to Three Years.* Philadelphia: Running Press, 1976. $4.95. This book presents ideas about having and raising children in a natural and supportive way. Includes a chapter on childbirth at home.

Emphasis on nutrition, breastfeeding, and family closeness.

Brook, Danae. *Naturebirth: You, Your Body, and Your Baby*. New York: Pantheon Books, 1976. $3.95. A lively book encouraging natural, fully conscious, family-oriented childbirth. By an English-woman.

Brooks, Tonya, and Linda Bennett. *Giving Birth at Home*. Cerritos, California: Association for Childbirth At Home, International, 1976. $6.00. Parent information handbook, spiral-bound, detailing aspects of preparation for home birth, labor guide, checklists for all stages, care of the newborn. Available with check or money order from the Association, ACHI National Office, Box 1219, Cerritos, California, 90701.

Caldeyro-Barcia, Roberto, M.D. "Some Consequences of Obstetrical Interference." *Birth and the Family Journal*, Vol. 2, No. 2 (Spring, 1975), pp. 34-38. This important article gives carefully detailed accounts of the hazards of the baby of induction and stimulation of labor.

Carroll, Robintree. "On Childbirth, Kids, and Love: An Interview with Ina May." *Well-Being*, No. 17 (Feb., 1977), pp. 28-35. This interview presents an overall portrait of midwifery at the Farm in Tennessee, including Farm views on childrearing, which are positive and sensible.

Chabon, Irwin, M.D. *Awake and Aware: Participation in Childbirth Through Psychoprophylaxis*. New York: Dell Publishing Co., Inc., 1966. $1.95. Good general work, focusing on the Lamaze technique, with historical perspective.

"The Childbirth Revolution," Special Report, *Harper's Weekly*, March 1- March 8, 1976, issue (Harper's Weekly, 2 Park Avenue, New York, New York 10016). Excellent issue; resources are listed, major trends in childbirth today are explored, many personal experiences are recounted.

Colman, Arthur, M.D., and Libby Colman. *Pregnancy: The Psychological Experience*. New York: Bantam Books, 1977. $1.95. First published by Seabury Press, 1971. Well-written book that discusses the stages of pregnancy and labor in the context of the feelings and experiences of expectant parents.

Committee on Perinatal Health. *Toward Improving the Outcome of Pregnancy: Recommendations for the Regional Development of Maternal and Perinatal Health Services* White Plains, New York: The National Foundation/March of Dimes, 1976. Report from a committee (of male obstetricians and pediatricians) in which a systematic approach is suggested to improve outcomes in maternity care through regional reorganization of facilities. An administrative look at the situation; remarkably little mention is made of the work of the nurse-midwife in obstetrical care, and consideration of the value of small obstetrical services is omitted.

Cox, Karen. "Midwives and Granny Women." Chapter in Wigginton, Eliot (ed.). *Foxfire 2*. Garden City, New York: Doubleday & Co., Inc., 1973. pp. 274-303. $4.50. A fascinating portrait of an American tradition of midwives, the rural grannies.

Davis, Adelle. *Let's Have Healthy Children*. New York: New American Library, $1.75. First published by Harcourt, Brace, and World, 1972. This book by the notable nutritionist gives good advice about diet during pregnancy.

Del Bo, L.M., M.D. *A Guide for the Future Mother*. Englewood Cliffs, New Jersey: Prentice-Hall, Inc., 1977. $4.95. Called "a practical medical manual on pregnancy, childbirth, and infant care," this book covers a wide range of material. Three of the chapters are devoted to Lamaze method, including a good physiological description of labor and delivery. The father's role is discussed also.

Dick-Read, Grantly, M.D. *Childbirth Without Fear: The Original Approach to Natural Childbirth*. New 4th Edition. New York: Harper & Row, Publishers Inc., 1972. Cloth, $10.95. Originally published 1944. Harper & Row Perennial Books Edition, 1976. $2.25. This is the basic text, Dr. Dick-Read's own theory and practice of natural childbirth.

Dick-Read, Grantly, M.D. *The Practice of Natural Childbirth*. Revised and edited by Helen Wessel and Harlan F. Ellis. New York: Harper & Row Publishers, Inc., 1970. $1.25. An abridgement of *Childbirth Without Fear: The Original Approach to Natural Childbirth*, new fourth Edition. This is the manual of Dick-Read's method; good information on breathing and relaxation and good description of labor and delivery.

Eastman, Nicholson J., M.D. *Expectant Motherhood*. 5th Edition. Boston: Little, Brown and Co., 1970. $2.75. A reasonable, standard introduction to pregnancy and birth, by a doctor.

Ehrenreich, Barbara, and Deirdre English. *Witches, Midwives, and Nurses: A History of Women Healers*. 2nd Edition. Glass Mountain Pamphlet No. 1. Old Westbury, New York: The Feminist Press, 1973. $1.95. A fascinating account of women healers in history and the persecution and suppression of them; political analysis with historical detail. As the authors say, "This pamplet represents a beginning of the research which will have to be done to recapture our history as health workers."

Eiger, Marvin S., M.D., and Sally W. Olds. *The Complete Book of*

Bréastfeeding. New York: Bantam Books, 1973. $1.50. First published by Workman Publishing Company, Inc., 1972. A standard, clearly written book on the subject.

Elkins, Valmai Howe. *The Rights of the Pregnant Parent*. New York: Two Continents Publishing Group, 1976. $4.95. Elkins expresses the need for a different kind of maternity care in terms of rights; it is a strong and careful book, with clear instructions: "How to get the childbirth you want" is the title of one section. Ms. Elkins organized the Montreal Childbirth Education Association.

Eloesser, Leo, Edith J. Galt, and Isabel Hemingway. *Pregnancy, Childbirth and the Newborn: A Manual for Rural Midwives*. 2nd English Edition. Mexico: Instituo Indigenista Interamericano, 1959. $3.50. Used to teach women prenatal care and how to deliver babies at home; written by midwives; an excellent basic book.

Ernst, Eunice K.M., and Mabel P. Forde. "Maternity Care: An Attempt at an Alternative." *Nursing Clinics of North America*, Vol. X, No. 2 (June, 1975), pp. 241-249. This article, available as a reprint from MCA (48 E. 92nd St., NYC 10028), describes the basic workings and philosophy of Booth Maternity Center in Philadelphia.

Ewy, Donna, and Rodger Ewy. *Preparation for Breastfeeding*. New York: Doubleday & Co., Inc., 1975. $2.95. Good, reassuring guide, emphasizes pyschological aspects.

Ewy, Donna, and Rodger Ewy. *Preparation for Childbirth*. New York: New American Library, 1974. $1.75. First published by Pruett Publishing Co., 1970. $5.50. Popular Lamaze guide.

Flowers, Charles. *Obstetric Analgesia and Anesthesia*. New York: Hoeber, Medical Division of Harper & Row, Publishers, Inc., 1967. Cloth, $10.00. A standard medical work on the subject; it supports preparation for childbearing.

Frazer, Sir James George. *The Golden Bough: A Study in Magic and Religion*. 1-Volume Abridged Edition. New York: The Macmillan Company, 1922. Source of multitudes of legends, facts, and myths; a popular early crosscultural work.

Gaskin, Stephen, and The Farm. *Hey Beatnik! This Is the Farm Book*. Summertown, Tennessee: The Book Publishing Company, 1974. $1.95. Story of how The Farm got started, with good descriptions of the beginnings of midwifery on The Farm, many birth stories, and very basic advice about delivering a baby.

Gelb, Barbara. *The ABC of Natural Childbirth*. New York: W. W. Norton & Co., Inc., 1954. A standard work, if one judges by the number of references to it in the literature. (No longer in print.)

Gioseffi, Daniela, and Esther Swartz. "Lifting the Veil of Isis."

Quest: A Feminist Quarterly, Vol. 3, No. 2 (Fall, 1976), pp. 70-76. This article explores the possibility that bellydancing has its origin in birth rituals.

Gold, Cybele, and E.J. Gold. *Joyous Childbirth: Manual for Conscious Natural Childbirth.* Berkeley, California: And/Or Press, 1977. $6.95. Emphasizes active participation of father. Preparation (physical and spiritual), the birth itself and communication with the newborn, and postpartum concerns are described and illustrated. There is also a coach's guide.

Gray, Henry. *Gray's Anatomy: The Illustrated Running Press Edition of The American Classic.* 1901 Edition. Philadelphia: Running Press, 1974. $8.95. Paperback edition of the famous anatomical work, clear and valuable. 1248 pages, a fine bargain.

Greenhill, J.P. and Emanuel A. Friedman, *Biological Principles and Modern Practice of Obstetrics.* Philadelphia: W.B. Saunders Co., 1974. This medical text goes back to 1913, *Principles and Practice of Obstetrics,* by Dr. Joseph B. DeLee, noted obstetrician.

Guttmacher, Alan F., M.D. *Pregnancy, Birth and Family Planning: A Guide for Expectant Parents in the 1970's.* New York: New American Library, 1971. $1.95. An updated version of a useful old standby; includes the conventional topics on pregnancy and hospital birth.

Haire, Doris B. *The Cultural Warping of Childbirth.* ICEA, 1972. $1.00. Originally published in Spring, 1972 edition of *ICEA News.* ICEA, PO Box 20852, Milwaukee, WI 53220. This pamphlet is the clearest and simplest presentation of the practices of standard American hospital obstetrics and the outcomes, in data form. Sobering information presented without any need for lengthy discussion. An important work. Doris Haire was president of ICEA from 1970 to 1972.

Haire, Doris B., and John Haire, *Implementing Family-Centered Maternity Care with a Central Nursery.* 3rd Edition. Hillside, New Jersey: ICEA, 1971. I haven't seen this, but *Our Bodies, Ourselves* describes it this way: "Complete guide for hospitals or anyone interested in converting a conventional maternity unit into a service where prepared mothers and fathers can participate fully in labor, delivery and care of the baby afterward. Exhaustive documentation."

Hallum, Jean L. *Midwifery.* New York: Arco Publishing Co., Inc., 1974. $5.00. As the introduction says, this book is a brief, easy-to-read textbook for midwives in training, by an Englishwoman. The emphasis is on childbirth as a natural phenomenon, though complications and interventions are discussed. Diagrams and drawings are numerous.

Harding, M. Esther. *Woman's Mysteries: Ancient and Modern*. New York: Harper & Row, Publishers, Inc., Harper Colophon Books, 1971. $3.95. A psychological interpretation of the feminine principles as portrayed in myth, story, and dreams—so reads the subtitle of this work, by a pupil of Carl Jung.

Hartman, Rhondda Evans, *Exercises for True Natural Childbirth*. New York: Harper and Row, Publishers, Inc., 1975. Cloth, $9.95. Childbirth preparation exercises for women; a companion book to Dr. Robert Bradley's *Husband-Coached Childbirth*.

Hazell, Lester Dessez. *Commonsense Childbirth*. New York: Berkley Publishing Corporation, a Berkley Medallion Book, 1976. $1.95. This is the general childbirth book that is most appreciated by expectant parents, in my experience. The author, past president of ICEA, writes clearly about the physiology of and the many possible choices in labor and delivery. The appendices are useful, the attitudes reassuring and fully informative.

Heardman, Helen. *A Way to Natural Childbirth: A Manual for Physiotherapists and Parents-To-Be*. 3rd Edition, revised and re-edited by Maria Ebner, Edingburgh: Churchill Livingstone, Medical Division of Longman Group Limited, 1974. $2.75. First written in 1948, this manual has been popular in England and here; Ms. Heardman did much to popularize the ideas of Dr. Read, and contributed interpretations of the value of specific relaxation techniques in childbirth preparation.

Hersey, Thomas. *The Midwife's Practical Directory*. 2nd Edition. Published by the author, Baltimore, 1836. Here included in reprint edition, New York: Arno Press Inc., 1974. Cloth, $18.00. (Part of series: *Sex, Marriage and Society*, Charles Rosenberg and Carroll Smith-Rosenberg, advisory editors) Interesting historically; strong on herbs and liniments.

Ina May, and The Farm Midwives. *Spiritual Midwifery*. Summertown, Tennessee: The Book Publishing Company, 1975. $5.95. A gorgeous, joyous book; the story of the kind of midwifery that grew at The Farm and grows there still; includes beautiful drawings and photos, numerous birth tales, and a practical manual of information on how to assist at births. A new edition of *Spiritual Midwifery*, published in late 1977, places greater emphasis on practical midwifery advice and has fewer birth stories than the first edition. The two are then a nice combination of editions to have.

Jacobson, Edmund. *How to Relax and Have Your Baby*. New York: McGraw-Hill Book Co., 1959. $3.95. Techniques of progressive relaxation applied to childbirth preparation, from the author of *Progressive Relaxation* (below), a work of importance in the history of the movement for natural childbirth.

Jacobson, Edmund. *Progressive Relaxation: A Physiological and Clinical Investigation of Muscular States and Their Significance in Psychology and Medical Practice.* 3rd Revised Edition. Chicago: University of Chicago Press, 1974. $18.00 (paper). First published in 1939. The original work on this subject, a technique formulated and reworked by Jacobson; his discovery was important to the natural childbirth movement in its beginnings, and has considerable relevance still.

Jones, Sandy. *Good Things for Babies.* Boston: Houghton Mifflin, 1976. $4.95. A superbly useful catalogue of items for babies, carefully chosen for safety, usefulness, and high quality. Clear photos, good tips on choosing, and first-rate bibliographies in several areas of childbearing.

Karmel, Marjorie. *Thank You, Dr. Lamaze: A Mother's Experiences in Painless Childbirth.* Garden City, New York: Doubleday & Co., Inc., Dolphin Books Edition, 1965. $1.95. First published by J.B. Lippincott Company, 1959. Personal and enthusiastic book; it provides an introduction for Americans to the theories and methods of Dr. Lamaze. Marjorie Karmel with Elisabeth Bing founded the American Society for Psychoprophylaxis in Obstetrics (ASPO) in 1960.

Kitzinger, Sheila. *The Experience of Childbirth.* 3rd Edition. Baltimore: Penguin Books Inc., 1972. $2.95. First published in Great Britain by Victor Gollancz, 1962. One of the best introductions to childbirth available. Kitzinger's style is marked by a refreshing concreteness; she always has a comparison to make that vividly expresses her point. Her techniques for natural childbirth, which she calls "psycho-sexual," include some excellent relaxation and massage suggestions, and she is enthusiastic about the importance of the husband in preparation and in labor. Kitzinger emphasizes the psychological aspects of pregnancy, labor, birth, and postpartum.

Kitzinger, Sheila. *Giving Birth: The Parent's Experience of Childbirth.* New York: Taplinger Publishing Co., 1971. Cloth, $7.50. A nice collection of accounts of personal experiences in childbirth, emphasizing the effects on the whole family.

Klaus, Marshall H., and John H. Kennell. *Maternal-Infant Bonding: The Impact of Early Separation or Loss on Family Development.* St. Louis, Missouri: The C.V. Mosby Company, 1976. $6.25. An excellent, important work, scholarly and precise without being hard to read. The authors, both professors of pediatrics, present the findings that show the importance of immediate physical contact between mother and newborn. The book also treats such questions as how to care for parents of premature, sick, or malformed infants, or of infants who die. Critical comments by other experts appear regularly in the text; interviews with parents are another valuable feature. The findings are extremely significant for obstetrical management.

Kroger, William S. *Childbirth with Hypnosis*. North Hollywood, California: Wilshire Publications, 1975. $2.00. An interesting presentation of the use of hypnotic techniques to counteract the pain of labor. The author tends to emphasize the need for an authoritarian physician to direct the entire experience; I found the book most useful in describing self-hypnosis.

La Leche League International. *The Womanly Art of Breastfeeding*. Franklin Park, Illinois: La Leche League International, 1963. $3.50. A classic work on the subject by the organization that for more than two decades has been offering instruction and support to nursing mothers. The information is solid and helpful; a *must* book for those planning to breastfeed, or for those simply interested in the subject.

Lamaze, Fernand. *Painless Childbirth: The Lamaze Method*. New York: Pocket Books, a division of Simon & Schuster, Inc., 1972. $1.95. Translation by L.R. Celestin, first published in the United States by Henry Regnery: Chicago, 1970. First published in English in Great Britain, 1958; first published in France, 1951. Dr. Lamaze's only book about the method that carries his name. This volume emphasizes the scientific background of Soviet psychology that produced the psychoprophylactic (later Lamaze) method. Includes Dr. Lamaze's own lectures. Dry and rather inaccessible.

Lang, Raven. *Birth Book*. Palo Alto, California: Science and Behavior Books/Genesis Press, 1972. $6.00. Raven Lang helped to establish the Birth Center at Santa Cruz, a noteworthy alternative birth choice in California from 1971 to 1974. There are some historical obstetrical data here, and some sound advice, but the accounts of home births and the remarkable photos of same are the heart of this interesting book.

Leboyer, Frederick. *Birth Without Violence*. New York: Alfred A. Knopf, Inc., 1975. $3.95 (Cloth $8.95). Original French edition entitled *Pour Une Naissance Sans Violence* (Paris: Editions du Seuill, 1974). A remarkable book by a French obstetrician who asks that we consider the feelings of the baby in arranging our birthgiving. Poetic and powerful, with remarkable photographs, including a series of a newborn put into a warm bath, smiling in amazement.

Leboyer, Frederick. *Loving Hands: The Traditional Indian Art of Baby Massage*. New York: Alfred A. Knopf, Inc., 1976. Cloth, $7.95. Like its predecessor, a lovely book, with photos that really match the text. The technique is presented clearly and simply, in the same gentle poetic style and with the same concerns as *Birth Without Violence*.

LeCron, Leslie M. *The Complete Guide to Hypnosis*. New York: Harper & Row, Publishers, Inc., 1971. $1.75. Includes a section on hypnosis in childbirth.

Lubic, Ruth Watson. "Nurse-Midwifery in Context." New York: Maternity Center Association. Reprinted from *Briefs*. A good, brief view of the history and place of nurse-midwifery in American obstetrics. This 12-page pamphlet is obtainable from MCA: 48 East 92nd Street, NYC 10028.

Lubic, Ruth Watson, and Eunice K.M Ernst. "Psychological Analgesia." From *Clinics in Obstetrics and Gynecology*, obtainable from MCA, $.50. A comprehensive review of methods of prepared childbirth.

Macfarlane, Aidan, M.D. *The Psychology of Childbirth*. Cambridge, Massachusetts: Harvard University Press, 1977. $2.95. An excellent concise exploration of some of the psychological aspects of birth: what is pain, how does the father feel, what is the nature of the sensitive period right after birth. The writing is particularly clear.

Magee, Joni, M.D. "Labor: What The Doctor Learns As a Patient." *The Female Patient*, Vol I, No. 11 (December, 1976), pp. 27-29. This article is most rare: a report from an obstetrician about how it feels to be on the receiving end of obstetrical care today. Sensitive and useful. Dr. Magee practices at Booth Maternity Center in Philadelphia.

Maternity Center Association. *A Baby Is Born*. 3rd Edition. New York: Grosset & Dunlap, 1964. Cloth, $5.95. Clear presentation of the phases of development; ideal text for family life courses and childbirth education. Photographs are of the famous Dickinson-Belskie sculpture series shown in *Birth Atlas*.

Maternity Center Association. *Birth Atlas*. New York: MCA. Sixth Edition, 1977. $20. Obtainable from MCA, 48 East 92nd Street, NYC 10028. Sculptor Abram Belskie, D.A., and Dr. Robert L. Dickinson, Designer and Draftsman, Modeler of Anatomy and Obstetrics, collaborated to produce sculptures depicting the unborn child, in various stages of embryonic and fetal development, in relation to the surrounding anatomical structures. Life-size sculptures of the baby during the progressive stages of labor form the core of this series, first displayed in 1939 at the World's Fair in New York. The *Birth Atlas*, spiral-bound, 14'' x 22'', offers superb photographs of these sculptures; also included are diagrammatic representations of the same. Complete and concise captions accompany each of the pictures. This handsome publication is used worldwide as a childbirth education aid.

Maternity Center Association. ''Birth Atlas Slide Series.'' New York: Maternity Center Association, 1973. Booklet accompanies 35-mm slides. $12.50 for 20 slides. Obtainable from MCA, 48 East 92nd Street, NYC 10028. Beautiful photos of the sculptures made for the 1939 World's Fair, depicting the progress of labor; the booklet is an excellent concise childbirth education course in itself.

Maternity Center Association. *Briefs: Footnotes on Maternity Care.* The official publication of Maternity Center Association. Ten issues per year. $4.00 per year. Write to MCA, 48 East 92nd Street, New York, New York, 10028. Excellent, up-to-date material in handy form.

Maternity Center Association. *Log: 1915-1975.* This nicely put together and illustrated pamphlet is not a commercially available product, but the history it presents is of considerable interest in looking at childbirth in 20th century United States.

Maternity Center Association. *Preparation for Childbearing.* 4th Edition. MCA, 1973. $1.00. First published, 1963. Excellent pamphlet, well illustrated; discusses comfort in pregnancy, participation in labor, and management of the postpartum period.

Maynard, Fredelle. ''Home Birth vs. Hospital Birth.'' *Woman's Day,* June 28, 1977. Presents the basic facts in the choice between these two modes of giving birth.

McCleary, Elliott H. *New Miracles of Childbirth: What Modern Medicine Is Doing to Make Childbearing Safer and Easier.* New York: Dell Publishing Co., Inc., 1974. $1.95. This readable book introduces some of the medical advances in obstetrics in recent years, such as the fetal heart monitor, surgery before birth, and life-saving techniques in premature births. The interview format is pleasant to read. McCleary also presents the case for paramedical, nursing, and nurse-midwife presence on the obstetrical team, in a positive and convincing way. Little, however, is included about the risks and contra-indications of the obstetric technology.

Mead, Margaret. *Blackberry Winter: My Earlier Years.* New York: William Morrow & Company, Inc., 1972. Cloth, $8.95. First volume of the autobiography of this remarkable anthropologist. Her writing is a model of clarity and interest.

Mead, Margaret, *Male and Female: A Study of the Sexes in a Changing World.* New York: William Morrow & Company, Inc., 1975. $4.95. First published 1949. Drawing upon decades of first-hand experience with several cultures, Dr. Mead leads us to and through some reflections and theories about the interactions of and similiarities and differences between male and female.

Medvin, Jeannine O'Brien. *Prenatal Yoga*. Albion, California: Freestone Publishing Co., 1974. $3.50. An attractive book which includes photographs of yoga postures that are appropriate and helpful for the pregnant woman. Spiritually inclined text.

Mehl, Lewis E., M.D., et al. "Home Birth Versus Hospital Birth: Comparisons of Outcomes of Matched Populations." Paper presented at 104th Annual Meeting, American Public Health Association, October, 1976. APHA, 1015 18th Street, NW, Washington, DC 20036.

Meltzer, David (ed). *Birth*. New York: Ballantine Books, 1973. $1.95. This book is a rare treat, a gathering from all over the world, from times ancient to modern, of legends and songs and poems and tales about birth; edited by a poet.

Milinaire, Caterine. *Birth*. New York: Crown Publishers, Inc., 1974. $5.95. A lively collection of personal stories, cultural lore from all over, preparation advice (including herbs and exercise), and physiological information.

Montagu, Ashley. *Life Before Birth*. New York: New American Library, 1964. $1.25. Covers ways in which the expectant mother affects the physical and emotional development of the child in utero.

Montagu, Ashley. *The Natural Superiorty of Women*. New York: The Macmillan Company, 1953. Revised Edition, 1974. $1.95. Interesting views of males and females; the section on men's envy of childbearing is quite unusual.

Montagu, Ashley. *Touching: The Human Significance of the Skin*. New York: Harper & Row, Publishers, Inc., Perennial Library edition, 1971. $2.95. A thoroughly fascinating work by the noted anthropologist, exploring our need for physical contact; supports the kinds of conclusions reached by Klaus and Kennell about the importance of physical touch in the forming of attachments between parents and new babies.

Mothering: Sharings on Natural Motherhood. Two issues per year. $6.00 per year. Vol. 1, July, 1976. Available from Box 184, Ridgway, Colorado, 81432. Articles, some in Spanish, about all aspects of "new" childbearing; poetry from parents, excellent bibliographies, and news from organizations like ICEA.

Myles, Margaret F. *Textbook for Midwives, with Modern Concepts of Obstetric and Neonatal Care*. Eighth Edition. New York: Churchill Livingstone, Division of Longman, Inc., 1975. $15.00 (paper). A practical text, thorough in obstetrical material, and also offering training in other midwife functions, such as prenatal education and instructions in "Parent-craft." Medical parts include descriptions of malformations and extensive detail about delivery. Excellent and technical; the miscellaneous sections include infertility, high-risk babies, and social aspects of obstetrics.

NAPSAC: *Safe Alternatives in Childbirth*. See under Steward, David, and Lee Steward.

Newton, Niles. *Maternal Emotions*. New York: Paul F. Hoeber, Inc., 1955. Out of print. This important early work is, unfortunately, hard to locate today; the kind of research that Ms. Newton continues to do directly treats psychological aspects of birth and the postpartum period, in particular the importance of establishing the right atmosphere.

Nilsson, Lennart, et al. *A Child Is Born*. New York: Delacorte Press, 1966. Cloth, $9.95. Dell paperback, 1977. $5.95. Completely Revised Edition, with "New photographs of life before birth and up-to-date advice for expectant parents," 1977. Cloth, $11.95. Originally published in Swedish, Stockholm: Albert Bonniers Forlag, 1965. Although this book includes a practical guide for the pregnant woman, its unique offering is the remarkable photographs of the fetus in utero as it develops, a wondrous achievement technically. The 1977 edition has new color plates and an updated text.

Noble, Elizabeth. *Essential Exercises for the Childbearing Year: A Guide to Health and Comfort Before and After Your Baby Is Born*. Boston: Houghton Mifflin Co., 1976. $4.95. This is a first-rate clearly written guide, full of extremely useful physiological information and attractive drawings. The chapter on Caesarean section is especially useful. Written by a physical therapist with a specialty in ob-gyn, it includes helpful daily advice for comfort during pregnancy and after birth.

Nofziger, Margaret. *A Cooperative Method of Natural Birth Control*. Summertown, Tennessee: The Book Publishing Company, 1976. $1.95. Clear and simple presentation of a combination method of determining when ovulation occurs and thus knowing when to refrain from intercourse. Emphasizes the responsible cooperation between the man and the woman.

Osol, Arthur, Chairman of Editorial Board. *Blakiston's Gould Medical Dictionary*. 2nd Edition. New York: McGraw-Hill Book Company, 1972. Detailed, precise, scientific. Gives word derivations; includes good color plates of systems of the body.

Our Bodies, Ourselves. 2nd Edition. See under Boston's Women's Health Book Collective, Inc.

Oxorn, Harry, and William R. Foote. *Human Labor and Birth*. 3rd Edition. New York: Appleton-Century-Crofts, 1975. $13.75 (paper). Basic textbook on normal obstetrics.

Planned Parenthood Federation of America, Inc. *11 Million Teenagers: What Can Be Done About the Epidemic of Adolescent Pregnancies in the United States*. A publication of the Alan Guttmacher Institute, The Research and Development Division of Planned Parenthood Federation of America, New York: Planned Parenthood, 1976. This is a model presentation, filled with facts and figures, well interpreted, well illustrated, compassionate.

Pritchard, Jack A., and Paul C. Macdonald. *Williams Obstetrics, Fifteenth Edition*. New York: Appleton-Century-Crofts, 1976. Cloth, $30.00. A standard obstetrical text whose new edition has more on fetal health and abortion than previous editions. The drawings and diagrams are very informative; references in each of the chapters are considerable; a promedication, pro-intervention attitude certainly occurs, but cautions are spelled out in most cases. The sections on disorders, diseases, infections, ruptures, and malformations are best left alone, I think.

Pryor, Karen. *Nursing Your Baby*. New York: Pocket Books, 1973. $1.50. First published by Harper and Row, 1963. Generally considered to be one of the best manuals on the subject.

Rich, Adrienne. *Of Woman Born: Motherhood As Experience and Institution*. New York: W.W. Norton & Company, Inc., 1976. Cloth, $6.95. Adrienne Rich, a major poet in America, combines her own experience as a mother with discussions of history, literature, and current events to provide this deeply thoughtful and provocative look at womanhood. Her writing is clear and powerful.

Rothman, Barbara Katz. "In Which a Sensible Woman Persuades Her Doctor, Her Family, and Her Friends to Help Her Give Birth at Home." *Ms.*, Vol V, No. 6 (December, 1976), pp. 25-32. Letters from the author to her sister provide a witty and descriptive look at the obstacles such a decision creates.

Sablosky, Ann H. "The Power of the Forceps: A Comparative Analysis of the Midwife—Historically and Today." *Women & Health*, Vol. 1 No. 1, (January/February, 1976), pp. 10-13. Sablosky's analysis of midwifery from a feminist perspective is lively and provocative, though brief; she emphasizes the strife between organized, male-dominated medical obstetrics and the popular lay tradition of midwifery. Her assumption that the Certified Nurse-Midwife will always practice only as an assistant to a doctor is, I think, unnecessarily pessimistic.

Salk, Lee. *Preparing for Parenthood*. New York: Bantam Books, 1975. $1.95. One of the best basic parenting how-to books, by the noted physician and child psychologist. He suggests the importance of and ways of arranging for the baby's arrival—preparing the home, working through feelings, helping the other children. Salk discusses birth itself, ways to make the most of a hospital stay, issues in infant feeding, and adjusting to life with a newborn.

Schaefer, George, M.D. *The Expectant Father: A Practical Guide,* Revised Edition. New York: Barnes & Noble Books, 1972. $2.25. First published by Simon & Schuster, 1964. Readable, practical advice for the father: how to get to the hospital on time, how to give support to the woman, how to prepare, how to evaluate drugs and procedures, how to figure costs. Best on psychological guidance; its technical information is too brief.

Seaman, Barbara, and Gideon Seaman, M.D. *Women and the Crisis in Sex Hormones.* New York: Rawson Associates Publishers, Inc., 1977. A large and thorough study, employing more than 8000 case histories, of what synthetic sex hormones do to human health. Included are such items as birth control pills, estrogen therapy for menopause symptoms, and DES (diethylstibestrol, the drug given to thousands of women in the 1950s to prevent miscarriage, now discovered to be the cause of vaginal and cervical cancer in the female offspring of these women and the cause of sterility in the male offspring). Ms. Seaman is the author of *The Doctor's Case Against the Pill* and *Free and Female.*

Shaw, Nancy Stoller. *Forced Labor: Maternity Care in the United States.* New York: Pergamon Press, Inc., 1974. $5.50. A fine sociological look at maternity care in the United States, based on close observation. Sparsely but well illustrated; academic and personal at the same time. May be hard to find in bookstores, except at universities. Shaw's suggestions about change in childbearing options are excellent.

Somer, Carol. "How Women Had Control of Their Lives and Lost It." *Second Wave,* 1972, pp. 5-10, 28. A brief history of midwifery from a feminist perspective.

Sousa, Marion. *Childbirth at Home.* New York: Bantam Books, 1977. $1.95. This is a sound, positive, responsible guide to the issues that will concern those who decide to give birth at home. Includes statistics from 300 home births in California.

Spiritual Midwifery. See under Ina May, and The Farm Midwives.

Spock, Benjamin, M.D. *Baby and Child Care.* Newly revised, updated, and enlarged (4th) edition. New York: Pocket Books, a division of Simon & Schuster, Inc., 1976. (First Pocket Book edition, 1946). $1.95. Still a bargain, and still a comfort; this edition reflects new information for our times, new emphasis on the participation of the father in child rearing, new awareness of changing roles for women; incoporates the findings of, for instance, Klaus and Kennell about maternal-infant bonding.

Stewart, David, and Lee Stewart. *Safe Alternatives in Childbirth.*

Chapel Hill, N.C.: NAPSAC, Inc., 1976. $5.00 plus $.50 shipping. This very important collection of articles provides summaries of opinions by midwives, obstetricians, nurse-midwives, and pediatricians about maternity services today; home birth and maternity center birth are emphasized as safe, practical alternatives to hospitals. The articles are exceptionally clear and concise, and many present good statistical information.

Tanzer, Deborah, and Jean Block. *Why Natural Childbirth*. New York: Schocken Books edition, 1976. $3.95. First published by Doubleday & Co., Inc., 1972. Tells the story of couples who shared birth in a "natural" way; from the experience of a psychologist.

Tucker, Tarvez. *Prepared Childbirth*. New Canaan, Connecticut: Tobey Publishing Co., Inc., The Women's Library, 1975. $2.95. This book presents in a plain and reasonable fashion the idea that childbirth is pleasanter and safer if the parents prepare themselves for the experience. Introduction by Elisabeth Bing, the noted Lamaze teacher.

Vellay, Pierre, M.D. *Childbirth with Confidence*. Translated by Eliot E. Philip. New York: The Macmillan Co., 1969. Cloth, $6.95. A good medical explanation of the psychoprophylactic (Lamaze) method, by Dr. Lamaze's colleague. This book is actually a guide to sexuality and reproduction as well as birth. The tone is dry and scientific. Dr. Vellay's attitude is unpleasantly patronizing at times, as when he refers to the laboring woman as a schoolgirl who has learned her lessons well, or badly; some others of his attitudes may strike the reader of today as prudish (using inappropriate slang such as "slit" for vagina).

Ward, Charlotte, and Fred Ward. *The Home Birth Book*. New York: Doubleday/Dolphin Books, 1977. $5.95. Revised edition of the book originally published by Inscape Corp., 1975. This book contains pieces written by doctors, midwives, parents, and child-birth educators about various aspects of home birth. Good blend of factual material and personal experience and good photos. Introduction by Ashley Montagu.

Wertz, Richard W., and Dorothy C. Wertz. *Lying-In: A History of Childbirth in America*. New York: Free Press/Macmillan, 1977. Cloth, $10. A serious look at the effects of the hospital way of childbirth in this country. The authors trace modes of giving birth from colonial times to the present and advocate a return to a less intervening approach.

White, Gregory J., M.D. *Emergency Childbirth: A Manual*. Franklin Park, Illinois: Police Training Foundation, 1958. Spiral-bound,

$4.00. Basic explanation of procedures for nonhospital deliveries, especially in emergency situations. Sensible and reassuring; simply and clearly presented. An important item to have if one is planning a home delivery.

Williams Obstetrics. See under Pritchard, Jack A., and Paul C. Macdonald.

Williams, Henry Smith, M.D. *Twilight Sleep: A Simple Account of New Discoveries in Painless Childbirth.* New York: Harper & Brothers, 1914. Out of print. An historical curiosity; hails scopolamine as a deliverer of women.

Williams, Phyllis, R.N. *Nourishing Your Unborn Child.* New York: Avon, 1974. $1.75. First published by Nash Publishing Company Corp., 1974. Balanced combination of the theoretical and the practical; straightforward and clear. In-depth discussion of nutritional values in food; sample menus included. Good preventive medicine.

Wingate, Peter. *The Penguin Medical Encyclopedia.* Baltimore: Penguin Books Inc., 1972. $3.95. A handy reference work, with historical as well as contemporary medical material. Treats obstetrical topics in some detail; the description of the course of labor is good, except that it fails to describe the particular character of transition.

The Womanly Art of Breastfeeding. See under La Leche League International.

Wright, Erna. *The New Childbirth.* New York: Pocket Books, 1971. $1.50. First published by Hart Publishing Company, Inc., 1967. Another fine English guide; Wright presents Lamaze technique interspersed with sound practical information about conception, pregnancy, labor, and delivery; includes helpful diagrams. Emphasizes importance of father.

Appendix

CHECKPOINTS FOR CONSUMERS OF FAMILY-ORIENTED OBSTETRICAL SERVICES

In choosing birth at home or at a maternity center, you may find a compatible attendant without much difficulty. If you are going to have your baby at a hospital, and you seek some variety of family-centered birth, the following points can help you select a situation that suits you. ICEA and La Leche League are widely available sources of referrals for names of doctors and hospitals who support natural, prepared childbirth. Friends, and friends of friends, can usually be counted on to give recommendations. Also, you can select names from the phone book. In your first visit with a doctor whom you are considering, keep in mind these questions. The same issues apply when you look at a prospective hospital, although this choice may be determined by your choice of obstetrician.

(1)—Is the husband welcome in prenatal care, labor, and delivery? Would another labor support person be welcome?

(2)—What standard medications, anesthetics, or procedures does the doctor/hospital use?

(3)—Does the doctor welcome your intention to prepare physically for birth?

(4)—Does the doctor/hospital electively induce labor?

(5)—Does the doctor routinely perform episiotomies?

(6)—Will the doctor support you if the hospital opposes practices of natural childbirth?

(7)—Will the doctor/hospital staff inform you and consult with you about administration of analgesics and anesthetics?

(8)—Will you be allowed to stay with your baby, assuming birth has occurred without mishap, and avoid routine separation after birth?

(9)—If it is a group-practice situation, do all the doctors share the same basic approach?

(10)—Does the doctor/hospital staff support breastfeeding? That is, not just not be opposed to it, but offer positive encouragement?

(11)—What is the doctor's/hospital standard procedure on position for labor and delivery? On routine shaving, enema, I.V.?

Many perfectly reasonable doctors might be put off by a barrage of pointed questions; you will be able to get a feel for the doctor's approach and personality after asking just a couple. Many of these details can be worked out in second and subsequent visits, once you have found someone you feel comfortable with. An attendant who offers only very quick visits each time and does not seem to want to go over with you your questions and fears and concerns may be too busy for the kind of childbirth experience you want.

LIST OF ABBREVIATIONS AND ACRONYMS

AAHCC	American Academy of Husband-Coached Childbirth
ACAH	Association for Childbirth at Home
ACHI	Association for Childbirth at Home, International
ACHO	American College of Home Obstetrics
ACNM	American College of Nurse-Midwives
ACOG	American College of Obstetrics and Gynecology
ASPO	American Society for Psychoprophylaxis in Obstetrics
BACE	Boston Association for Childbirth Education
CbC	Childbearing Center (MCA)
CEA	Childbirth Education Association
CMC	Chicago Maternity Center
CNM	Certified Nurse-Midwife
C/SEC	Caesareans/Support, Education, and Concern
fhm	fetal heart monitor
FNS	Frontier Nursing Service
GP	general practitioner
HOME	Home Oriented Maternity Experience
ICEA	International Childbirth Education Association
I.V.	intravenous
LLLI	La Leche League International
MCA	Maternity Center Association
MCEA	Montreal Childbirth Education Association
NAPSAC	National Association of Parents and Professionals for Safe Alternatives in Childbirth
ob/gyn	obstetrics/gynecology
RDS	respiratory distress syndrome

RN	registered nurse
SACH	Safe Alternative Childbirth at Home
SPUN	Society for the Protection of the Unborn Through Nutrition

ELY'S TABLE OF THE DURATION OF PREGNANCY

Explanation: In the upper horizontal row of numbers, find the date of last menstruation; the number beneath, set in *italics*, will show the expiration of 280 days or ten months of 28 days each.

	1	2	3	4	5	6	7	8	9	10	11	12	13	14	15	16	17	18	19	20	21	22	23	24	25	26	27	28	29	30	31	
January	1	2	3	4	5	6	7	8	9	10	11	12	13	14	15	16	17	18	19	20	21	22	23	24	25	26	27	28	29	30	31	
October	*8*	*9*	*10*	*11*	*12*	*13*	*14*	*15*	*16*	*17*	*18*	*19*	*20*	*21*	*22*	*23*	*24*	*25*	*26*	*27*	*28*	*29*	*30*	*31*	*1*	*2*	*3*	*4*	*5*	*6*	*7*	*November*
February	1	2	3	4	5	6	7	8	9	10	11	12	13	14	15	16	17	18	19	20	21	22	23	24	25	26	27	28				
November	*8*	*9*	*10*	*11*	*12*	*13*	*14*	*15*	*16*	*17*	*18*	*19*	*20*	*21*	*22*	*23*	*24*	*25*	*26*	*27*	*28*	*29*	*30*	*1*	*2*	*3*	*4*	*5*				*December*
March	1	2	3	4	5	6	7	8	9	10	11	12	13	14	15	16	17	18	19	20	21	22	23	24	25	26	27	28	29	30	31	
December	*6*	*7*	*8*	*9*	*10*	*11*	*12*	*13*	*14*	*15*	*16*	*17*	*18*	*19*	*20*	*21*	*22*	*23*	*24*	*25*	*26*	*27*	*28*	*29*	*30*	*31*	*1*	*2*	*3*	*4*	*5*	*January*
April	1	2	3	4	5	6	7	8	9	10	11	12	13	14	15	16	17	18	19	20	21	22	23	24	25	26	27	28	29	30		
January	*6*	*7*	*8*	*9*	*10*	*11*	*12*	*13*	*14*	*15*	*16*	*17*	*18*	*19*	*20*	*21*	*22*	*23*	*24*	*25*	*26*	*27*	*28*	*29*	*30*	*31*	*1*	*2*	*3*	*4*		*February*
May	1	2	3	4	5	6	7	8	9	10	11	12	13	14	15	16	17	18	19	20	21	22	23	24	25	26	27	28	29	30	31	
February	*5*	*6*	*7*	*8*	*9*	*10*	*11*	*12*	*13*	*14*	*15*	*16*	*17*	*18*	*19*	*20*	*21*	*22*	*23*	*24*	*25*	*26*	*27*	*28*	*1*	*2*	*3*	*4*	*5*	*6*	*7*	*March*
June	1	2	3	4	5	6	7	8	9	10	11	12	13	14	15	16	17	18	19	20	21	22	23	24	25	26	27	28	29	30		
March	*8*	*9*	*10*	*11*	*12*	*13*	*14*	*15*	*16*	*17*	*18*	*19*	*20*	*21*	*22*	*23*	*24*	*25*	*26*	*27*	*28*	*29*	*30*	*31*	*1*	*2*	*3*	*4*	*5*	*6*		*April*
July	1	2	3	4	5	6	7	8	9	10	11	12	13	14	15	16	17	18	19	20	21	22	23	24	25	26	27	28	29	30	31	
April	*7*	*8*	*9*	*10*	*11*	*12*	*13*	*14*	*15*	*16*	*17*	*18*	*19*	*20*	*21*	*22*	*23*	*24*	*25*	*26*	*27*	*28*	*29*	*30*	*1*	*2*	*3*	*4*	*5*	*6*	*7*	*May*
August	1	2	3	4	5	6	7	8	9	10	11	12	13	14	15	16	17	18	19	20	21	22	23	24	25	26	27	28	29	30	31	
May	*8*	*9*	*10*	*11*	*12*	*13*	*14*	*15*	*16*	*17*	*18*	*19*	*20*	*21*	*22*	*23*	*24*	*25*	*26*	*27*	*28*	*29*	*30*	*31*	*1*	*2*	*3*	*4*	*5*	*6*	*7*	*June*
September	1	2	3	4	5	6	7	8	9	10	11	12	13	14	15	16	17	18	19	20	21	22	23	24	25	26	27	28	29	30		
June	*8*	*9*	*10*	*11*	*12*	*13*	*14*	*15*	*16*	*17*	*18*	*19*	*20*	*21*	*22*	*23*	*24*	*25*	*26*	*27*	*28*	*29*	*30*	*1*	*2*	*3*	*4*	*5*	*6*	*7*		*July*
October	1	2	3	4	5	6	7	8	9	10	11	12	13	14	15	16	17	18	19	20	21	22	23	24	25	26	27	28	29	30	31	
July	*8*	*9*	*10*	*11*	*12*	*13*	*14*	*15*	*16*	*17*	*18*	*19*	*20*	*21*	*22*	*23*	*24*	*25*	*26*	*27*	*28*	*29*	*30*	*31*	*1*	*2*	*3*	*4*	*5*	*6*	*7*	*August*
November	1	2	3	4	5	6	7	8	9	10	11	12	13	14	15	16	17	18	19	20	21	22	23	24	25	26	27	28	29	30		
August	*8*	*9*	*10*	*11*	*12*	*13*	*14*	*15*	*16*	*17*	*18*	*19*	*20*	*21*	*22*	*23*	*24*	*25*	*26*	*27*	*28*	*29*	*30*	*31*	*1*	*2*	*3*	*4*	*5*	*6*		*September*
December	1	2	3	4	5	6	7	8	9	10	11	12	13	14	15	16	17	18	19	20	21	22	23	24	25	26	27	28	29	30	31	
September	*7*	*8*	*9*	*10*	*11*	*12*	*13*	*14*	*15*	*16*	*17*	*18*	*19*	*20*	*21*	*22*	*23*	*24*	*25*	*26*	*27*	*28*	*29*	*30*	*1*	*2*	*3*	*4*	*5*	*6*	*7*	*October*

Index

The Author Speaks

I set about the task of writing The Birth Primer as an investigative reporter: to read articles and books, yes, but also to talk, question, observe, listen. Visits to hospitals, maternity centers, and home settings, including The Farm in Tennessee, showed me much that the literature could not. I attended prenatal classes at Booth; watched childbirth education films; went to lectures; talked with midwives and doctors; corresponded with writers and childbirth educators; and visited with pregnant and just-delivered friends, collecting birth stories from anyone who had them. I watched as two babies were born.

I met weekly with Dr. John Franklin at Booth Maternity Center, questioning him about obstetrics, hearing from him what various segments of the obstetrical community were doing and thinking these days. He gave me a sense of where change is coming and expanded my sense of the issues. Dr. Franklin read the manuscript, corrected factual materials, and kindly opened the doors at Booth for me. I thank him for his involvement. Any remaining inaccuracies are my own.

To Susannah May, who makes me a mother for sure: I thank her for her loving support, for her being herself.

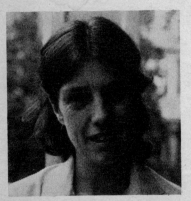

Rebecca Parfitt works as a writer, focusing in particular on maternity issues, women's employment, and arts of Japan. She graduated from Swarthmore College in 1964, has worked in film and video, and has taught English in addition to being a freelance writer. Originally from New Hampshire, she now lives in Philadelphia with her daughter, who is ten.

SIGNET Child Care Books for Your Reference

☐ **JOYOUS CHILDBIRTH: Manual for Conscious Natural Childbirth by Dr. Cybele Gold and Dr. E. J. Gold.** Clear and complete instructions for childbirth with minimum artificial intervention, including a complete guide and list of supplies for childbirth at home. "The best of Lamaze and Leboyer . . . recommended!"—*Human Behavior*　　(#E8122—$2.25)

☐ **THE MOTHERS' AND FATHERS' MEDICAL ENCYCLOPEDIA by Virginia E. Pomeranz, M.D., and Dodi Schultz.** From infancy through adolescence, an all-inclusive reference book designed to give you fast, accurate, and vital information when you need it most. Fully illustrated.　　(#E7779—$2.50)

☐ **THE NEW AMERICAN MEDICAL DICTIONARY AND HEALTH MANUAL by Robert E. Rothenberg, M.D., F.A.C.S.** This revised third edition includes a complete Medicare Handbook and up-to-date information on contraceptive drugs and devices in addition to over 8,700 definitions of medical terms, diseases, and disorders, a comprehensive health manual with a first-aid section, charts and tables on diets, obstetrics, child development, and much, much more. With over 300 illustrations.　　(#E8314—$2.50)

☐ **LIFE BEFORE BIRTH by Ashley Montague.** Revised and edited. Vital information for the mother-to-be to increase her chances of bearing a normal, healthy baby. Introduction by Dr. Alan F. Guttmacher.　　(#E9184—$2.25)

☐ **RAISING THE ONLY CHILD by Dr. Murray Kappleman.** Clear and direct prescriptions for raising a healthy only child from infancy to young adulthood, exploring such potential problems as isolation and loneliness, peer relationships, insecurities and dependency problems, and much more.　　(#J8501—$1.95)

Buy them at your local

bookstore or use coupon

on next page for ordering.

SIGNET Books You'll Want to Read

Ⓟ